Chronic Fatigue

Other books in this series:

Angina
Arthritis
Asthma
Depression
Diabetes
High Blood Pressure
How to Stop Smoking

Coming soon:

How to Stay Healthy
Menopause

Chronic Fatigue

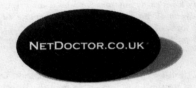

Series Editor
Dr Dan Rutherford

Hodder & Stoughton
LONDON SYDNEY AUCKLAND

The material in this book is in no way intended to replace professional medical care or attention by a qualified practitioner. The materials in this book cannot and should not be used as a basis for diagnosis or choice of treatment.

Copyright © 2003 by NetDoctor.co.uk
Illustrations copyright © 2003 by Amanda Williams

First published in Great Britain in 2003

The right of NetDoctor.co.uk to be identified as the Author of the Work has been asserted by them in accordance with the Copyright, Designs and Patents Act 1988.

10 9 8 7 6 5 4 3 2

British Library Cataloguing in Publication Data
A record for this book is available from the British Library

ISBN 0 340 86138 X

Typeset in Garamond by Avon DataSet Ltd,
Bidford-on-Avon, Warwickshire

Printed and bound in Great Britain by
Bookmarque Ltd., Croydon, Surrey

The paper and board used in this paperback are natural recyclable products made from wood grown in sustainable forests. The manufacturing processes conform to the environmental regulations of the country of origin.

Hodder & Stoughton
A Division of Hodder Headline Ltd
338 Euston Road
London NW1 3BH
www.madaboutbooks.com

Contents

Foreword

All over the world, for no apparent reason, people have been falling sick with a mystery illness which seems to puzzle doctors and patients alike. Young healthy people, most often women in their teens and twenties, find that they are suddenly extremely tired, have pain all over their bodies and have sleep disturbance and inexplicable problems such as memory loss. They go to their doctors and after the usual time delay – 'must be some kind of a virus' – they have blood tests and referrals, only to be told that 'there is nothing physically wrong'. Not surprisingly such a verdict has a profoundly depressing effect on these people and their families, and they are often driven to despair not only by the lack of a diagnosis but by the fact that they cannot continue to hold down a job or to look after their families.

Researchers from all over the world have agreed that there are common criteria for this illness and that it can have a name. In the United Kingdom it has been called ME, in France spasmophilia, in the US CFIDS. Community-based studies have shown that it is one of the commonest women's health problems in modern societies and that it has a profound effect on the health and wellbeing of families and young children whose mothers and sometimes fathers are afflicted. The researchers have preferred the term CFS but for the purposes of this book we will call it CFS/ME. Naming the illness and affirming the person has been of great benefit to those who find themselves in this medical mystery and the key issue is recognition of this very important syndrome and recognition of the suffering and bravery of those who have to endure its very distressing symptoms.

This book sets out to explain in simple terms what is involved in this process of recognition and clearly describes all aspects of professional care from listening to the presentation to excluding other possible causes or diagnoses, to the principles of symptom control. The relationship between the physician and the person with CFS/ME is absolutely central to the management of this condition and no book can substitute for the support and care of an ongoing therapeutic relationship. However, the CFS/ME patient has problems in this area. Too often he or she is dismissed as a 'heartsink patient', an unfortunate term which describes the state of the doctor and not the patient. Doctors all over the world declare their belief, or not, in the problem and finding a sympathetic and professional attitude can be difficult. Furthermore the symptoms of poor memory and concentration mean that, even when these rare qualities are present, the person leaves the doctor without any clear recall of what was said.

This book will be a valuable reference to help people and their families at all stages of this difficult illness find their way out of a series of difficult problems. It describes with clarity and a great deal of common sense many of the pitfalls of the illness and its treatment. Above all, it is full of hope, and rightly so, because the majority of sufferers eventually recover and discover that there is life after CFS/ME. Unfortunately there are also a small number who never find that respite but even for them it will be comfort to know that the problem can be looked at as logical, understandable and the substance of an agenda which can be discussed with sceptical and unbelieving doctors. I would thoroughly recommend it for people with CFS/ME and their families and, above all, for their doctors.

Professor J. Campbell Murdoch MD, PhD, FRCGP, FRNZCGP,
FRACGP, FACRRM
Head of the School of Primary, Aboriginal and Rural Health Care
University of Western Australia

Acknowledgements

Generally speaking, people with chronic fatigue syndrome/myalgic encephalomyelitis (CFS/ME) have been poorly served by the medical profession. There are notable exceptions and Professor Campbell Murdoch is one of them. A pioneer in research and management of chronic fatigue syndrome, previously a family doctor in New Zealand, Professor and Chair of the Department of General Practice in Dunedin School of Medicine and now Professor and Head of the Rural Clinical School at the University of Western Australia, he still found the time to review this book. His own book *Chronic Fatigue Syndrome: A patient-centred approach* (Radcliffe Medical Press), written with colleague and ex-patient Harriet Denz-Penhey, was an invaluable source of information and inspiration. It should be required reading for all doctors, not just those who look after people with CFS/ME, dealing as it does with the essence of treating someone who is ill. Patients too will find it a rewarding and informative read.

Special thanks are always due to the editorial team at Hodder and Stoughton, notably Julie Hatherall for this volume.

Although great care is taken to ensure the accuracy of the information in the NetDoctor book series I remain responsible for any errors. Suggestions on how the content can be improved are also welcome. Please send any comments to me at d.rutherford@netdoctor.co.uk

Dr Dan Rutherford
Medical Director
www.netdoctor.co.uk

Chapter 1

The Problem of 'Fatigue'

Introduction

Most of this book is concerned with the condition known as chronic fatigue syndrome, or myalgic encephalomyelitis (ME). Right away there is a difficulty in giving an adequate name to this condition that satisfies the various forms it takes and encompasses the often profound impact it can have on an affected individual. As yet a totally satisfactory name does not exist, for reasons that will become clear shortly. As a compromise we'll use the hybrid term 'CFS/ME'.

Terms

'Chronic' is often used in common speech to mean 'terrible' or 'rubbish' but it is the medical term for long-lasting and has no other medical meaning. 'Syndrome' means a pattern of symptoms and clinical findings that together form a recognisable picture of an illness but for which the cause is unknown, or in which several causes might be possible but result in the same pattern of illness.

'Myalgia' means painful muscles, which is a common feature of CFS/ME but 'encephalomyelitis' means 'inflammation of the brain and nerves', which in a strict sense has not been demonstrated to occur in CFS/ME. To this extent, therefore, the term ME is inaccurate but has been left until a better alternative is proposed.

Fatigue itself is a very common feeling that occurs in a host of circumstances, sometimes as a symptom of illness, at other times as an emotion or as a reaction to life events. The scope for confusion in the medical use of the word fatigue is fully realised in practice, and has considerably added to the difficulties experienced by people who have CFS/ME, and indeed those who care for them. We'll try to dispel this confusion by considering fatigue in a wider sense too.

What's in a name?

The importance of giving a name to a condition far exceeds the convenience of needing fewer words to refer to it. A name means a diagnosis, or at least it does within the confines of Western medical thinking. Under this system not having a name is equivalent to not existing at all, and for many people affected by CFS/ME their consequent contact with medical services has indeed been as if they had a purely imaginary illness. As we'll make clear, these days of ignorance are rapidly being left behind but significant numbers of badly informed health professionals continue to under-serve people with CFS/ME, and the facilities available to sufferers are often poor or absent. Fortunately the drive for improvement has come from the highest levels within the Health Department in the UK, joining at last the reasonable and well-argued case put forward over many years by the CFS/ME support organisations and charities. A major report commissioned by the

Chief Medical Officer for England, published in 2002, endorsed the acceptance of CFS/ME as a real and disabling illness that badly needs proper research and the provision of adequate facilities and support. The Scottish Executive agreed with these findings in February 2003 (see appendix A for references).

The future for people with CFS/ME is at least beginning to look up. Not yet, admittedly, in terms of a more exact understanding of the condition or in the arrival of curative treatments but certainly in attitudes and approaches to management. CFS/ME does not yet have an ideal name, but it does at last have credibility in the minds of those health professionals deserving of the title. We'll return later to the important issue of the nature and the quality of the care currently provided to people with CFS/ME, and the implications arising from it.

What is fatigue?

A dictionary or thesaurus will give several alternative words or phrases such as weariness, exhaustion, tiredness or lack of energy but we all know from our own experience what it means to be 'fatigued'. In normal circumstances the feeling of physical tiredness is related quite obviously to a cause such as excess effort. It may be enough to force us to rest but it then improves in a short time. Repeated physical effort tends to improve our fitness and ability to carry out heavy or sustained work. Mental fatigue is equally familiar to anyone who has tried to cram for an examination, or remember important information after a night without adequate sleep. We can get 'fatigued' just from being bored of having nothing to do.

Fatigue is often linked to our mood and is a common symptom in depression. It may be the primary reason for someone with unrecognised depression to go to the doctor. The relationship and importance of fatigue to mood is often misunderstood by patient and carer alike, and has given rise to some of the largest areas of dissatisfaction felt by people with CFS/ME. It is explored further in chapter 2.

The severity and impact of the symptoms experienced by the majority of people with CFS/ME is vastly greater than the symptoms of what one might call 'ordinary' fatigue, which is one of the reasons that the term 'chronic fatigue syndrome' fails to convey an adequate picture of the condition as far as some people who have it are concerned. There is usually a delay of anything from hours to days between the effort and the exhaustion in CFS/ME and repeated activity does not lead to adaptation and improvement in strength or stamina – usually the reverse occurs. Clearly these features distinguish the fatigue of CFS/ME as an altogether more substantial and pervasive feeling than that which is within the ordinary experience of most people.

Although fatigue is a central feature of CFS/ME, and it is the logical place to start in considering the condition, it is not necessarily the most important feature of the illness in a particular person. The other aspects of CFS/ME and diagnosing the condition properly are covered in more detail in chapter 2.

The size of the problem

It is no exaggeration to say that CFS/ME is a major world-wide public health problem. There are considerable difficulties in establishing good figures for the number of people affected because of differences in the criteria used for making a diagnosis (and the acceptance of the illness as a diagnosable one by many doctors), in the effectiveness of the methods used to gather statistics about the condition, in the accuracy of such statistics in accounting for ethnic groups and the differences between countries with different health care systems.

Accepting that the figures are approximate, the following generalisations can be made regarding the UK:

- CFS/ME affects between two and four people per 1000 of the population.

- It affects people of all ages, including children as young as five years old.
- The commonest age of onset is between the early twenties to mid-forties.
- CFS/ME is diagnosed about twice as often in women compared to men.
- It affects all social classes.

There are therefore as many as 200,000 people with CFS/ME in the UK alone – a staggering number for a condition that has attracted so little serious enquiry until recently. Some surveys in fact put the potential number as higher than this, so it should be seen as a conservative estimate.

Understanding fatigue

There are ways to explain at least some aspects of general fatigue within the knowledge that we already possess about how our bodies work. Having some appreciation of these processes is useful when considering how CFS/ME might come about. Perhaps one of the most valuable outcomes of such an exercise is the realisation of how little we know of the precise way in which nerves, muscles and brain work together. Lack of a healthy respect for one's own ignorance is a fault common to many practitioners who have difficulty dealing with CFS/ME, believing their own knowledge of human function to be so complete that they can confidently deny the existence of the condition.

NERVES
Nerve cells exist by the million within the brain and throughout the spinal cord. Multiple nerve fibres extend from each cell and connect up in highly complex ways between themselves and with

5

other tissues such as muscle, hormone-producing glands, the digestive system and other internal organs. In the brain the nerve cells are largely arranged on the surface of the organ, which is folded to increase its surface area. This is the 'grey matter' of the brain, whereas the interconnecting nerve fibres underneath are the 'white matter'. Many of the nerve connections within the brain link different parts of the brain together, whereas others connect to nerve cells down the length of the spinal cord, which in turn run through larger nerves to the other tissues.

The number of possible ways that brain cells can link up is incredibly high – there are said to be more possibilities than the number of atoms in the entire universe. Signals travelling between brain cells make up the basic way in which we think, see, hear, imagine, feel, memorise, recall and feel emotion and so on. The complexity of the process is so great that we are only just beginning to understand it.

Although brain cells and nerves are a bit like electrical cables and switches in the way they pass signals around they in fact use a combination of electrical impulses and chemical reactions to deliver their messages to each other. Where a nerve fibre reaches another nerve cell to which it is connected the fibre ending spreads out to form a highly specialised connection zone – the 'synapse'. Here the fibre ending and the cell are very close to each other, but do not actually touch. The scale of an individual nerve connection is extremely small – of the order of a few thousandths of a millimetre across.

Within the nerve ending there are microscopic 'packets' of a particular chemical compound held in readiness. Upon the arrival of the signal at the nerve ending the nerve releases tiny amounts of this signalling chemical into the gap between it and the surface of the next cell. The chemical crosses the gap and links with receptor molecules on the other cell's surface. These receptors are specifically shaped proteins that 'recognise' the signalling chemical just as a lock recognises the correct key. When that happens the signal to the cell is triggered.

Further chemical reactions then occur which destroy the signalling chemical at the nerve cell surface, so freeing the receptor in readiness for the next signal to be received. Also, the end of the first nerve takes back any free chemical that has not been used up in the signalling process. A similar process is used throughout the nervous system – for example when a nerve sends a signal to a muscle fibre, telling it to contract.

Through its many connections each nerve cell is therefore in touch with a great many others, and therefore can potentially receive large numbers of signals at any one time. However, not all incoming signals switch the receiving cell to the 'on' state – many act in the opposite direction to make the cell less likely to be triggered. Therefore it is the balance between 'on' and 'off' signals that determines what the result will be for an individual cell. This seems to be the basic way in which the huge diversity of brain function arises – subtle changes in the patterns of activity in some cells have knock-on effects on other cells, which in turn change events in other parts of the brain.

This scheme of nerve signalling, called synaptic transmission, has been very well studied and is undoubtedly accurate. As a result of this knowledge it has also been possible to design a whole range of drugs that act in specific and largely predictable ways. For example, modern antidepressant drugs boost the effect within the brain of some messenger chemicals, such as serotonin, which are known to be depleted in depression.

The observed reactions in synaptic transmission also provide some explanations for the process of fatigue. It will be clear that only so much messenger chemical can be present at any one time and that once the supply is exhausted it will be impossible for a signal to cross that synapse until the stores of messenger chemicals have been re-built. This is known to happen in normal nerve function. It is also known that the nerve receiving the signal becomes increasingly insensitive to stimulation the more it is stimulated. Experts in this branch of biology call this 'synaptic fatigue'. After a break, which is usually quite short, the constant manufacturing process within nerve endings re-stocks the supplies of messenger chemical so that further signals can be passed on. Similarly the sensitivity of the receiving cell quickly returns to normal.

MUSCLES

A similar picture is observed within muscle tissue. Muscle can contract because of the unique shapes of the two types of protein molecule that it is made of (actin and myosin). These interlink in a similar way to your fingers when slid together. In the relaxed state just the 'fingertips' are meshed, but when signalled to contract the 'fingers' slide fully home. Multiplied millions of times this gives sufficient power to move limbs and body. Several mechanisms cause muscles to fatigue, one of which is that the energy-supplying molecules within the muscle cells become used up more quickly than they can be replaced. Second, the sensitivity of the muscle cell to the incoming nerve signal drops off, so decreasing the effect of the nerve stimulation. Third, a tensely contracting muscle blocks off the supply of blood coming into it, and without blood (and therefore oxygen) it cannot sustain its activity.

Relevance to CFS/ME

Abnormalities of synaptic transmission or muscle function at the molecular level have not been found in CFS/ME, so you may be wondering what is the purpose of the preceding biology lesson. This is an important issue, because even well-intentioned doctors, who do believe their patients, can find this a sticking point too.

What these theories do not explain is what drives the motivation to carry out an act such as a muscle movement, or how it is that we can move one muscle and not its neighbour just by thinking about it. A mechanical explanation of how nerves interact explains precisely nothing about the phenomenon of memory, or the function of sleep, or what makes the difference between clear thinking and confusion. The signals we can detect from electrodes stuck into muscles do not explain how movement is co-ordinated for a purpose, or why two people can be so completely different in the skills they possess, or what makes someone a brilliant pianist.

This is information that we don't have, and perhaps we never will, but a moment's thought clearly shows that even the most powerful microscope or sophisticated scanner can give us only a fraction of the answers we need to truly understand the processes of life. Furthermore, mind and body must be totally integrated in complex living beings such as us. People who consider illness (or health for that matter) in terms of being either 'mental' or 'physical' are using a concept that is good only for a kindergarten level of understanding of human biology and behaviour. It is not good enough for a professional approach to the care of ill people. Patients expect more than this from their doctors and other health carers who in turn ought to require higher standards of their own knowledge.

In chapter 3 we will mention some of the research findings that have been discovered in CFS/ME. It is as yet a jigsaw puzzle with only a few pieces available, and no picture on the box to go by. For the meantime the most important concept to accept is that CFS/ME operates at a more subtle level than can be demonstrated with present medical technology. Undoubtedly the mists surrounding the condition will blow away in time but our current level of understanding does not allow us to get close enough to the mechanisms involved. This should not matter, as the same is true of a great many other conditions that are accepted and treated within conventional medicine. For example, although much is known about the immune system we don't know what makes some people develop immune-system problems such as allergic disease whereas others do not. We know little of the brain chemistry changes that cause schizophrenia, yet no one denies it exists or avoids trying to treat it. We know that smoking clogs up people's arteries but not exactly how it all happens. There are endless examples of medical conditions for which we have little or no understanding of the disease processes causing them. That does not make them less important.

The professionally mature doctor or nurse sees the person that is the patient. They do not see 'cases'. Acceptance of the ill person for what they are is the starting point for any successful relationship between him or her and a carer. CFS/ME has unfortunately proved to be one of the best examples of how such relationships can go wrong, largely because of neglect of this fundamental principle of good medical care.

The purpose of this book is to help people with chronic fatigue. Lengthy criticism of medical services and attitudes won't advance that cause without some suggestions of how to improve the situation. It's also important to put the inadequacies of the medical provision for CFS/ME to date into context. Although there will always be dinosaur thinkers in every walk of life, including medicine, there are many more people involved in providing care to people with CFS/ME who want to help their patients but are unsure of the facts about the condition and consequently don't quite know what to do for the best. We'll therefore return to these topics in later chapters.

SUMMARY

- Chronic fatigue syndrome and myalgic encephalomyelitis are unsatisfactory terms for the same condition. Presently the term CFS/ME is accepted as a compromise.
- CFS/ME is now properly recognised by the UK Department of Health as a real and disabling condition for which improved medical services are necessary.
- At least 200,000 people in the UK, from all walks of life and almost all age groups, are affected by CFS/ME.
- Precise explanations for the processes that underlie CFS/ME are lacking.

- Complete explanations of any illness are beyond present medical and scientific knowledge, but this should not prevent patients from receiving good care.

Chapter 2

Defining and Diagnosing Fatigue

The origins of CFS/ME

The terms chronic fatigue syndrome and myalgic encephalomyelitis have arisen in the past few decades but the condition to which they refer is unlikely to be new, any more than an orchid is new when first discovered and named. However, the illness we now recognise as CFS/ME was first described in nurses working during an epidemic of polio in Los Angeles in 1934. Several more occurrences of the illness occurred over ensuing decades across the world, usually involving people working within institutions, notably hospitals. Nearly 10 per cent of the medical and nursing staff of the Royal Free Hospital in London were affected in the famous episode of 1957, and for years afterwards 'Royal Free Disease' was another term in common use for this condition.

Definitions

In chapter 1 we alluded to the difficulties that occur when a disease is ill defined and lacking an agreed name. From the point of view of conducting research on a condition it is essential that agreement exists on what it is that is being studied, or conclusions made in one centre will have no relevance to anywhere else. Several groups around the world have therefore worked to produce definitions of CFS/ME that attempt to encapsulate the necessary features of the condition. The most widely used are those of the Centre for Disease Control (CDC, 1994) in the USA, which are:

- Fatigue of definite or new onset that is not the result of exertion, is not significantly improved by sleep or rest and which results in substantial reduction in overall performance for a consecutive period of six months or longer.

Plus at least four from this list:

- Self-reported significant impairment of short-term memory or concentration.
- Sore throat.
- Tender lymph glands (small swellings under the skin which are part of the immune system) in the neck region or under the armpits.
- Muscle pain.
- Headaches of a new type, pattern or severity.
- Unrefreshing sleep.
- Malaise following effort that lasts more than 24 hours.
- Pains in several joints occurring without joint swelling or redness.

Medical diagnosis is never so simple that it can be reduced to ticking off points on a list, and there are several problems using a system like this. For a start the requirement for the fatigue to be present for six months takes no account of the fact that the disability from CFS/ME starts on day one of the illness, which is often abrupt. In practice no caring doctor would wave a patient out of the consulting room and ask them to make an appointment once the six months were up so that he could then start discussing the symptoms for real.

In the early weeks of CFS/ME it can be difficult or impossible to distinguish it from other conditions that can cause similar symptoms but which have a different outcome, and it is necessary to search for these. Even so, should there be a reasonable suspicion that CFS/ME is the cause of someone's illness then it can and should be discussed early on. Even if someone does not have a full house of symptoms it would be very likely that a doctor who was sufficiently aware of CFS/ME would be willing and able to make a confident diagnosis of it once the initial medical assessment was complete and the results of some simple tests were confirmed normal. The purpose of these diagnostic criteria therefore should be seen as mainly an aid to research. People who fulfil them are therefore similar at least to a certain extent, so it becomes possible to compare how they fare with different types of treatment. It is quite possible to have CFS/ME and not have all of these symptoms – an individual's experience of CFS/ME is essentially unique.

International criteria

There are also some differences in the diagnostic criteria that have been developed in different countries, although they are not fundamentally different to the CDC list. Those from New Zealand and the UK, for example, place no importance on the presence of a sore throat or tender lymph nodes in diagnosing CFS/ME. The inclusion of these points in the CDC list harks back to earlier theories of the cause of CFS/ME that gave prominence to viral infection, notably glandular fever in which both these features are common. However, sore throat or lymph nodes would not be commonly associated with CFS/ME in those patients seen in the UK.

The 'Oxford Criteria' (1990) therefore defined CFS/ME as a syndrome in which:

- there is a definite onset (i.e. it is not lifelong);
- fatigue is the main symptom;
- the fatigue is severe, disabling and affects both physical and mental functioning;
- the fatigue has been present for at least six months, during which time it has been present more than 50 per cent of the time;
- other symptoms may be present, particularly myalgia, mood and sleep disturbance.

Tests

In making a diagnosis of CFS/ME it is important to exclude other conditions that can cause some or all of the symptoms, although there are really no other conditions that look exactly like it in all its aspects. Fatigue of a generally smaller degree is, however, a common accompaniment of anaemia (low haemoglobin), under-activity of the thyroid gland, diabetes, disturbance of kidney or liver function and persistent infection, especially with some viruses and more unusual bacterial infections. Rarer causes include immune system diseases such as lymphoma, 'auto-immune' diseases such as SLE (systemic lupus erythematosus) in which many organs become inflamed, or under-production of hormones from the pituitary gland of the brain. Simple blood and urine tests can screen for the majority of these conditions and are well within the scope of the GP to arrange. It is very uncommon for an alternative cause to remain undiscovered after someone has been through a reasonably thorough medical examination and these other tests but doubt may still be present in a proportion of people. Then the GP needs the help of a specialist, preferably one with a special interest in CFS/ME. These are very few in number anywhere in the UK, so patients may sometimes be seen by physicians who have no more knowledge of CFS/ME than their GP.

In the majority of people who have CFS/ME it will, however, be possible to make a positive diagnosis of the condition based on its own features, in which case these extra tests help to confirm that nothing else has been missed. An unhelpful line of thinking among 'dinosaur doctors' is to say to a fatigued patient, on receipt of a normal set of blood reports, that there is 'nothing wrong'. To the patient sitting in the chair and feeling completely whacked by the effort of getting to the surgery nothing could be more obviously wrong with such a view.

The availability of sophisticated blood tests, scanners and other types of modern investigation has bred an overly technical attitude towards diagnosis in some doctors. If they can't see a cause on a laboratory report, then they can't make a diagnosis or offer sensible advice on management. In the days not so long ago when there were fewer technical aids available, doctors relied more on their basic skills of history taking and clinical assessment and would rarely be stuck for a diagnosis upon which the patient could then act. Perhaps that diagnosis was less often correct in an academic sense than it could be now, but it was less likely to leave the patient high and dry with nothing to go on.

The high-tech aspects of modern medicine are of course very valuable when sensibly applied but we have to constantly remember that even with the best of our technology we get no more than a glimpse of the workings of our own biology. A full blood screen will have lots of numbers on it but it is still only a fuzzy picture seen from a distance of a world of complexity. To use an analogy, our current image of what makes us tick is equivalent to a view of the moon through a high-powered telescope. We can see far more detail than we can with the naked eye but much less than an astronaut walking on the surface inspecting individual grains of moon dust.

Put simply, one can diagnose very few things on tests alone. It is essential for the doctor to accept that the patient has come to the consultation because he or she feels ill, and that is the position from which the healing process has to start. A 'scientific diagnosis', apart from being mostly an illusory concept based on over-simplified thinking, must never be seen as an admission ticket without which the patient can't be offered help.

Many doctors, including some holding high academic office and with no doubt the best intentions, continue to struggle with the concept of illness for which they cannot find a positive test. They have even given it an official name – 'persistent unexplained physical symptoms' or 'PUPS'. The implications of this are explored later in the book.

Mental health

If you agree with the concept that mind and body are inextricably linked then you should find it easy to see why it is essential to take account of a person's mental well-being in any illness, not just CFS/ME. This is an area where there has been much misinformation and prejudice around and in the following section we'll try to clarify any misunderstandings.

Mood disturbance such as depression is very common in the general population, with at least one person in five developing a significant depressive illness at some point in their lives. The true figure is probably higher as depression, and mental illness in general, are conditions we don't like to talk about much, or admit to having. Even the term 'mental illness' is one with dark connotations. 'Mental' is often used in slang to mean 'deranged' or 'violent' or some other unsavoury meaning. The term 'illness' tends to imply that the depressed person is sick, or necessarily needs treatment – and probably with drugs. Such ideas are often wrong – for example, many people successfully get over depression without any need for drug therapy – but a fear that admitting the symptoms of depression to a doctor will lead to a label of psychiatric illness puts many people off seeking help. Of particular importance to someone with CFS/ME is the common observation that depression can take many different forms. It often appears as a physical illness first, perhaps of profound fatigue or a loss of weight, and in fact shares many symptoms in common with CFS/ME in addition to fatigue, such as impaired concentration and memory and sleep disturbance.

Distinguishing depression from CFS/ME

This is where the stumbling block lies. Some people with CFS/ME are also depressed, whether as a result of being unwell or, equally likely, because those factors that can cause CFS/ME are the same as those that can cause depression. It's unclear whether people with CFS/ME are any more likely to become depressed than the average for the population – some studies have suggested so but others have shown the same incidence.

What is clear is that many people with CFS/ME find it insulting to have a diagnosis of depression given to them and many doctors close their minds to treating people with CFS/ME by deciding that it is a psychiatric condition. Neither position is justified, for several reasons.

The first is that depression is a real condition too, just as is CFS/ME. It causes real disability and does not deserve to be taken as a second-class or undesirable diagnosis. As a society we've got to get rid of the stigma attached to depression, and the best way to do that is to cast out individual prejudices concerning mental illness in general. Second, the features of a true depressive illness are not the same as those of CFS/ME when considered as a whole. People with CFS/ME who are not truly depressed will not express feelings of guilt, or a diminished sense of pleasure in life, nor will they harbour suicidal ideas, all of which are classic symptoms of depression. It really should not pose any difficulty to distinguish these two illnesses except when they are mild, when the similarities are stronger. Third, although there is good evidence that brain chemistry disturbances occur in depression, which gives modern antidepressant medication its rationale for being used, the level of knowledge we have about these chemical abnormalities comes nowhere near explaining the whole condition. Antidepressant drugs are often very effective but they still have to be seen as crude tools working on a very fine mechanism. Much of what goes on in depression is just as mysterious and unexplained as the processes of CFS/ME. Given that fact it is surely not difficult to accept that there are probably common abnormalities in both conditions that account for the overlap between them.

When depression is detected, it needs to be treated effectively. It is very unlikely that any progress will be made with co-existing CFS/ME until this is done, so a doctor is well justified in pursuing a diagnosis of depression. At times it will be difficult to dogmatically say that some degree of depression is or is not present. In those circumstances it is reasonable for the doctor to suggest a trial of antidepressant medicine in case it helps. Antidepressant treatment otherwise has only a limited place in CFS/ME (see chapter 5).

Impact of CFS/ME

If you are reading this as someone who has or had CFS/ME you will need no expansion on the subject of how dramatic and devastating its impact can be. Although it is part of the diagnostic criteria for CFS/ME that it should significantly impair performance intellectually and socially, these few words hardly do justice to just how much CFS/ME can change someone's life. The level of impairment caused by CFS/ME can vary from fairly modest, in which an affected person can retain the ability to carry out most normal duties including work, provided this is paced and sufficient rest is allowed for, through to the most severely affected people who can be bed bound and need total nursing care. CFS/ME can last for months or even many years.

The knock-on effects of such a change in a person's abilities are of course far reaching. They can compromise employment, lead to financial difficulty, strain personal relationships and cause secondary ill health such as depression. There can be difficulties in accessing health care, not just in finding a sympathetic carer (although that hopefully is getting easier) but for those whose mobility is impaired there are transport problems getting to appointments and the effort of doing so can be just too much.

Ongoing uncertainty surrounding CFS/ME disheartens people who are already unwell and can make them defensive or reluctant to seek the help they need. The early experience of someone with new-onset CFS/ME in their contact with health services can be critical in shaping their subsequent dealings with those who are meant to help them. Although many receive positive and supportive advice from the start, those who don't can find themselves lost. The CFS/ME support organisations have been the only useful source of help for too many people with CFS/ME, and this needs to change.

SUMMARY

- Fatigue is one of the commonest symptoms experienced by people and seen by doctors.
- Fatigue is a central feature of CFS/ME and is usually more profound and longer lasting than fatigue from other causes.
- There are several other features of CFS/ME apart from fatigue and the combination makes the condition recognisable and diagnosable in its own right.
- The 'official' criteria for diagnosing CFS/ME are largely there for research purposes. In practice it is possible to diagnose CFS/ME with fewer features present.
- Tests to detect other possible causes of overlapping symptoms are part of good medical practice when someone first develops CFS/ME.

- Depression and other forms of mood disturbance are common in the general population and people with CFS/ME are not immune to being also affected.
- Depression can be positively diagnosed, and responds to treatment.
- CFS/ME can have profound and far-reaching consequences for the individual affected. The unpredictability and variable length of time the illness lasts emphasise the need for understanding and sympathetic support, which may have to extend over many years.

Chapter 3

The Causes of CFS/ME

We've already alluded to the fact that an all-encompassing explanation of what causes CFS/ME has not yet been found. Many experts and sufferers also believe that CFS/ME should be thought of as an umbrella term for a group of illnesses that are very similar, thus accounting for the variation in the patterns and severity of CFS/ME observed in different people. It certainly seems to be the case that CFS/ME is a destination that can be reached by different roads.

It is now well accepted that many illnesses develop when an individual who has a susceptibility to a condition then meets a set of circumstances that brings that tendency to the surface. Diabetes, several forms of arthritis, high blood pressure, asthma and other allergic diseases are just a few of the conditions in which the tendency is probably built into a person's genes. If some other trigger factor comes along, which could be a viral infection, environmental exposure to a toxic substance or drug or an emotional event, then a chain reaction is set off that leads to the illness.

Even in conditions which have been intensely studied we know of only a few genetic 'markers' which, if present, will definitely increase someone's risk of developing a particular disease. This is an area in which knowledge is expanding fast and concepts will undoubtedly change significantly over the next few years.

However, this is not to say that we have no idea at all what can cause CFS/ME. There are lots of little bits of information that contribute some degree of understanding. Also, some theories that have held sway for a time have subsequently been shown to be inaccurate.

Virus infection

Viruses are nearly the smallest of all living organisms, comprising little more than a bundle of genetic information (RNA or DNA) in a protein coat. Viruses cannot survive on their own – they have to get inside a living cell where they then hitch a ride using the cell's own biochemical processes for duplication of the virus material. A virus therefore gets right to the core of the host cell and it's easy to see why virus infection can have such powerful effects on an infected person.

One of the commonest ways in which CFS/ME is observed to come about is following a virus infection. Usually this will be a 'flu'-like illness associated, therefore, with a lot of general upset such as muscle aches, fever and fatigue. Only this time, instead of lasting two to three weeks, the person fails to recover and goes on feeling as if they have flu all the time. Post-viral fatigue syndrome is another of the terms that have been applied to CFS/ME in the past.

Virus infection would have also explained the pattern of CFS/ME as it was observed in the early episodes described in the literature, in which it occurred in minor epidemics, usually within closed com- munities such as hospitals that would have facilitated spread of an infectious cause. Such a pattern is, however, not now seen and most people who develop CFS/ME do so in isolation, with no other affected people around them.

Upper airway virus infections such as the common cold do not seem able to trigger CFS/ME but much attention has been focused on several other specific viruses over the years as possibly the main culprits. Polio virus, Epstein Barr virus (a cause of glandular fever), measles virus, viruses causing gastroenteritis and others have all at some time been under scrutiny but none has been consistently linked with the illness. Polio virus infection is now virtually unseen in the developed world as it is effectively prevented by immunisation but a small proportion of people who had polio in the mid-twentieth century develop what is called post-polio syndrome decades later. This has many features in common with CFS/ME but is not due to reactivation of the polio virus. Instead it is due to late damage of nerve and muscle tissue initially triggered by polio virus. Possibly, therefore, a similar mechanism could explain CFS/ME in some people.

In the course of normal recovery from most viral infections the virus is eliminated from infected cells. This is, however, not true of all virus infections. Shingles, for example, is due to reactivation of the virus that causes chickenpox, which, after a chickenpox infection, remains in the body forever within the roots of the nerves near the spinal cord. Although persistence of virus infection has not been proved in CFS/ME there are some experts who remain of the opinion that this is one way the condition may arise. In this theory the genetic materials of the viruses become incorporated into the host's own DNA and alter the function of the infected cells but they do not otherwise leave any mark of their presence and so are impossible to detect.

Immune system

Again, no consistent patterns are found but several research studies have found some alterations in the function of the immune system in people with CFS/ME. The immune system itself is a very complex and widely distributed collection of cells and tissues throughout the body. The lymph nodes are one component and are linked by a system of conducting tubes that in turn feed into the bloodstream. Within the lymph nodes, and dispersed throughout the blood and other tissues, are different members of the cell populations that make up the immune system. Some of these are designed to detect invaders such as foreign proteins, bacteria and viruses and others are capable of destroying foreign materials. Yet others can recruit more immune system cells to the site of infection by sending out chemical signals. Linkages between the immune system and other cells in the nervous system and in hormone-producing glands are all part of this highly sophisticated network. Thus infection can lead to immune reactions and hormone and nervous system changes, which together cause the symptoms such as fatigue, muscle pains or mood change.

Some studies have shown increased numbers of detector cells and circulating chemical signalling compounds, indicating an increase in alertness of the immune system in CFS/ME but also poorer function of the scavenger cells, indicating inefficiency of the clearance mechanisms. The changes are not marked and they tend to wax and wane, but neither are they normal.

Nervous system

Most attention has focused on the role in CFS/ME of the regulatory functions of the brain. The hypothalamus is the name given to the small central brain structure that acts as our master control unit, monitoring and adjusting body temperature, appetite, sleep, blood pressure, thirst and hormone balance. The hypothalamus is extensively connected to other brain regions and also to the pituitary gland directly below it – it's the 'spaghetti junction' of the brain's signalling system. The pituitary gland is about the size of a pea but, like the hypothalamus, its size belies its great importance. It produces a range of controlling hormones, which in turn stimulate the production of thyroid hormone, sex hormones and the body's natural steroid hormones. Other pituitary hormones influence the release of insulin from the pancreas gland (which controls the level of glucose in the blood) and another controls the production of urine from the kidney. The pituitary gland is controlled mainly by nerve signals coming down from the hypothalamus above as well as by hormones released by the hypothalamus into a tiny network of blood vessels connecting the pituitary and hypothalamus together.

It is easy to see how important are the hypothalamus and pituitary gland and to appreciate that disturbance in their function will potentially have marked knock-on effects in the body. However it is very difficult to conduct research on them. These structures are deep within and below the brain, well out of the reach of probes and sampling devices, even if these were safe things to use. Perhaps because of the technical difficulties such tests of hypothalamic function as do exist have shown conflicting results in CFS/ME. Some have shown a loss of some aspects of the automatic controls it normally carries out and others have not. Nonetheless many experts feel that the hypothalamus is where the problem lies in CFS/ME. This would explain why so many of the standard medical tests are normal in this condition but until we have better ways to test the hypothalamus then this theory cannot be proved.

Psychological illness

We've made the point already that mind and body are integrated, not separate, and that a fair view of any illness needs to take this into account. Considering only 'physical' causes of CFS/ME, such as virus infection or immune system abnormality, will therefore give an incomplete picture and it is essential to consider the psychological aspects too. Entrenched views that CFS/ME is due either to some outside influence or 'all in the mind' lead to dead-end arguments that do not help people with the condition.

Proponents of the 'all in the mind' camp are generally health professionals following standard medical reasoning and to an extent this is understandable. No one denies the existence of anxiety states, phobias, hysteria and similar conditions that are within the sphere of psychological illness. These are very real conditions that can disrupt a person's life severely but which are amenable to psychological treatment. Similarly, although we understand little of what causes schizophrenia or depression this doesn't stop us diagnosing and treating people who are affected. For none of these conditions is there a blood test or a scan – the diagnosis is made by speaking to someone and observing their behaviour, and matching the pattern to those that have been recognised and accepted over the years and written down in textbooks and disease classification systems.

The important point here is that a psychological or psychiatric diagnosis is not an end point in itself. It gives a name to an observed type of behaviour, but it does not explain it. However, because doctors and psychologists are trained to recognise these patterns, which are described in detail in the classifications of disease, there is an overwhelming compulsion for them to stop thinking any further when they have made a psychological diagnosis. Of course we can't wait for the complete answer to why illnesses occur before we treat them – to do so would mean no illness could be treated – so from a practical point of view making a psychological diagnosis allows treatment to start that has been found by experience to be helpful in other people who have the same diagnosis. So if in some people with CFS/ME psychological therapy seems to help, then well and good, it should be used. But what shouldn't happen, and too often does, is that a diagnosis of psychological illness is taken to be the end of the story. Some further examples will illustrate the point.

In recent years other conditions equally perplexing to medical science have come along, such as Sick Building Syndrome, Gulf

War Syndrome, Irritable Bowel Syndrome and Multiple Chemical Sensitivity. Those who favour a one-sided view of illness class these conditions as 'functional somatic syndromes', meaning illnesses that show themselves as physical but which have no 'organic' basis, i.e. all the tests are normal. This of course assumes that the tests we have available are sufficiently clever and sensitive to detect any possible abnormality – which is not the case. Some believe these conditions are powered by a system of false beliefs and worries on the part of the sufferer. Among those beliefs are erroneous concerns about being seriously unwell and destined to get worse, the positive effects of adopting the 'sick role' and possibly some interest in compensation and litigation. These undertones seem to creep through the assumptions made by those who are willing to diagnose CFS/ME as a psychological condition and feel that having done so, there is no need to go any further.

However, as we've just pointed out, a psychological diagnosis is no more than a recognised pattern of behaviour. It has no fundamental scientific basis, so when a doctor says that an illness in which all the tests are normal must be a psychological one he is only substituting one form of uncertainty with another. It really is a very shaky way to think, but doctors do it time and again because of the way in which they are taught to work.

From the patient's point of view too there can be misconceptions about what psychological illness is about. It tends to be seen as the second division of illness, something that means you aren't actually all that ill, or that you are making it up. Such ideas can be fuelled by misinformed media coverage and, it has to be said, by some health professionals too.

Hopefully we've made the case for a more sensible way to think about the psychological aspects of CFS/ME (or any illness). There is always a psychological dimension to being unwell and it needs to be taken into account in the healing process. The degree to which this dimension plays a part is entirely individual to the person affected and is unrelated to what might be the root cause of the condition. The psychological impact of illness is real and should not be underestimated as it may be the predominant factor in keeping an illness going. Considering CFS/ME to be 'only a psychological condition' is superficial and blinkered thinking.

It seems clear that there are many possible causative factors in CFS/ME, and equally clear that there is a large amount of research waiting to be done on this important illness. It is lamentable that so many question marks still hang over the condition, which has been quite neglected by mainstream medicine. However, as we'll cover in the next chapter, attitudes are now changing towards acceptance and enquiry rather than dismissal.

Predisposing factors for CFS/ME

It is a plausible idea that some people may be more prone than others to develop CFS/ME, particularly as this is true of many other illnesses. Females are about twice as likely as males to be affected and, although it is unknown why this should be, there could be a link with female sex hormones and their release from the ovaries, which is a process controlled by other hormones released from the pituitary gland and the hypothalamus of the brain.

There is a slightly greater likelihood of CFS/ME occurring in other members of the same family but it is not known whether this is because of a genetic tendency that they share, or because they are in close proximity and exposed to similar environmental influences.

No consistent findings have emerged from studies that looked at the personality types of people with CFS/ME. The 'yuppie flu' label of the 90s was completely inappropriate. There is also no definite evidence that having a history of previous mental ill health makes people any more likely to develop CFS/ME. It is possible though that someone with a past history of depression will suffer a relapse should they become chronically ill from another reason, such as CFS/ME.

Trigger factors

Predisposing factors may set the dominoes on end but a trigger factor is needed to knock the first one over. We covered infections at the beginning of this chapter and a history of a flu-like illness or gut infection is the most likely one to turn up at the beginning of someone's CFS/ME illness, but even so this is only in a minority of people. Immunisations could conceivably play a similar role to infection in triggering a reaction that leads to CFS/ME, but there is no proof that this happens. The benefits of immunisation certainly exceed any theoretical risk of getting CFS/ME.

'Stress' is notoriously difficult to measure but major life events such as bereavement, divorce and redundancy are undoubtedly stressful and are well known to be associated with triggering mood disturbance. Some people with CFS/ME can relate the onset to a stressful period in their own life.

Toxins have been proposed as a possible trigger for CFS/ME, particularly organophosphate pesticides. These are certainly known to be toxic to nerve tissue but there is no established link between them and CFS/ME. However, a long delay in onset of illness following the exposure to a toxin can make any link hard to prove, or to detect. Botulism is a form of food poisoning caused by a bacterial toxin that can paralyse muscles. It occurs in improperly canned foods and has occurred in rare outbreaks in the UK, one of which happened in 1989 in Lancashire and Wales. Survivors were followed up and some developed CFS/ME in subsequent years although there was no correlation between doing so and the severity of the poisoning.

Pregnancy can be a time when CFS/ME symptoms improve, but there may be a rebound worsening after the birth.

Maintaining factors

A mixed bag of factors can potentially prolong or exacerbate the disability of CFS/ME and it therefore makes sense to minimise those that are modifiable. If stress at work is a major issue then a period off work is sensible. For most people not in jobs with protected sick pay prolonged leave usually leads to some financial hardship with an increase in stress, so it can be counterproductive. As CFS/ME can arise over a short period of time in someone used to working hard, there can be a strong compulsion to force oneself to carry on at the usual pace. That is usually not a successful strategy and can lead to more symptoms and longer recovery. But accepting disability is not easy and can lead to anxiety over the future and depression if the CFS/ME carries on, as it often does, for a very long time.

Just as too much effort can be harmful, so can too little. Unused muscles get weak and a loss of fitness adds to fatigue. Sleep disturbance, a main feature of CFS/ME, is itself very tiring and saps one's mental energies. It's clear that there are many conflicts in an illness like CFS/ME, which can only be resolved by an individually tailored programme of management that is sensitive to change. It needs to take advantage of good spells but not push ahead too forcefully, while trying to minimise the disruption when disability is greater. A sympathetic and supportive home environment is essential, but not always present. Caring for someone with severe CFS/ME can put a strain on relationships. A lack of professional support can be particularly damaging.

Belief systems concerning the cause and consequences of CFS/ME can themselves prove to be obstacles to care. We've mentioned the problems that arise from a split physical/psychological mindset and how this can lead to conflict between those who are ill and those who look after them.

Strategies that can be used to treat CFS/ME are outlined in chapters 5 and 6. Before getting there, some issues concerning the medical approach to CFS/ME to date need to be aired.

SUMMARY

- No single cause of CFS/ME has been found and it is more likely that several causes exist that can trigger the illness in susceptible individuals.
- It is impossible to predict in advance an individual's likelihood of developing CFS/ME. It can happen to anyone.
- There is supportive evidence for the role of virus and bacterial infections, immune system abnormalities, environmental toxins and disturbance of hormone control and of the regulatory functions of the brain in the causes of CFS/ME.
- The psychological aspects of CFS/ME are significant but do not explain why the condition occurs.
- The course of CFS/ME is unique to the affected individual and requires a tailored management programme.
- Most of all someone with CFS/ME needs to be accepted as an ill person and not a 'case'.

Chapter 4

CFS/ME and the Medical Profession

Several times in the preceding chapters we've mentioned examples of the relationship between people with CFS/ME and health professionals not being a happy one. The purpose of this book is to help CFS/ME sufferers and not to be a sounding board for dissatisfaction, but many of the surveys of the experiences of those who've had CFS/ME confirm that there is a need for change in some professional attitudes. There are also positive messages that need to be emphasised, as not everyone is doing a bad job of looking after people with CFS/ME. It therefore seems appropriate to give this matter some space.

Chief Medical Officer's Report, 2002

In 1998 Sir Kenneth Calman, then Chief Medical Officer for England, said:

> I recognise Chronic Fatigue Syndrome is a real entity. It is distressing, debilitating and affects a very large number of people. It poses a significant challenge to the medical profession.

Later that year his successor, Professor Sir Liam Donaldson, set up a Working Party on CFS/ME which published its report in January 2002 (see appendix A for web links). This was an excellent and comprehensive report, which, although not solving issues such as the causes of CFS/ME, did clearly state the deficiencies in care that exist presently for sufferers. It also made several recommendations for change, which were endorsed by the Department of Health. These included: the need for health and social care professionals to accept that CFS/ME is a chronic illness; a request to the Medical Research Council to establish a strategy for research into CFS/ME; that recommendations to professionals on best management should be developed and integrated with others dealing with long-term disability; and that patients should become part of this process of change through the Government's 'expert patient' programme. A year later the Scottish Executive confirmed its acceptance of these proposals for Scotland. Leaving aside the inordinate amount of time it took for these documents to become reality, and the lack of pledged funds to enable them to work, any sufferer of CFS/ME might fairly ask why it was necessary to go to such lengths in the first place. Why has it taken so long for doctors to believe their patients?

The doctor-centred doctor

CFS/ME has exposed the failings of standard Western medical training more than almost any other condition. Doctors who are able to brilliantly diagnose and treat someone with advanced heart disease or complex chest problems can prove themselves useless in dealing with CFS/ME if they do not have the capacity to see the person before the patient. Western medicine depends on a diagnosis like a car depends on the ignition key. Without the right diagnosis, you can't make a start, and without any diagnosis at all you are stranded. Too much faith in technical aids and laboratory tests have convinced the Western doctor that either a) you can't be unwell if all the tests are normal or b) if all the tests are normal and you are still unwell then you must have a mental illness.

The modern doctor has come to assume the central role in deciding when someone is or is not ill. This is the doctor-centred approach and it's used because it works. Not always for the benefit of the patient, but it works for the medical system, which is overloaded and under-staffed. Using a doctor-centred approach puts the doctor in command of the consultation, allowing him or her to set the agenda for the questions that get asked, and to interpret the answers selectively. Thus it is possible to quickly see someone who is complaining of lower tummy pain on passing urine, prescribe an antibiotic for a presumed infection and move on to the next patient. On the day that might indeed be all that is needed to deal with that particular problem. It will certainly not be the only problem the patient has in her life, but it might be the only one she wants to deal with that day, so this may be quite a successful consultation.

If instead this lady ('Jill') comes in complaining of a headache sometimes when she passes urine, the consultation will not go so quickly. The doctor is unable to easily think of a medical condition that causes headache on passing urine, so he would probably try first to reassure Jill that it can't be serious. He checks Jill's blood pressure, which very rarely has anything to do with headaches, but it makes him feel he's covering all the options and he feels it's likely to further reassure Jill. Her blood pressure is perfectly normal. Clutching at straws a bit for a physical explanation for the symptoms he offers to check her urine just in case and asks her to come back in a couple of weeks if the problem isn't going away. However, Jill insists that the headaches are severe when they happen and she's worried about them. Now this doctor is on less certain ground. Unable to make a firm diagnosis he's already wondering if Jill is psychologically unwell. He's also getting flustered because several extra patients have been added to his already busy surgery list (he can see this on the computer on his desk) and he feels the time pressure building. He reasserts his control of the consultation, prescribes a painkiller to tide Jill over and asks her to come back the next week if she doesn't get any better. Realising she won't get any further that day Jill leaves and goes to the appointment desk.

This was not a good consultation. Jill herself felt that it was odd she should sometimes get headaches on passing urine, but she knew it was sore when it happened and persisted long enough to cause her a lot of trouble. She wanted the doctor to offer an explanation and was disappointed that he didn't seem to take her very seriously. He was pleasant but seemed in a hurry to get her out of the room.

At the appointment desk Doctor A, whom she's just seen, is in fact booked up for the next week and then is off on holiday, so she accepts an appointment with Doctor B although she hasn't met him before.

The patient-centred doctor

Next week Jill has an hour's wait before Doctor B calls her into his consulting room as he's running behind time. She explains about the headaches and that she'd handed in a urine sample (which is normal) and is relieved to see that he is interested, although he admits that he can't immediately explain the symptoms. However, he asks how they are bothering her and so she explains about them and that sometimes she dreads going to the toilet in case she gets another headache. He doesn't ask very many questions but sits back in his chair and listens attentively to what she has to say. At one point Jill mentions that she's worried she's keeping him back but he smiles and tells her not to worry about that at all, and that he wants to hear her whole story. After 20 minutes they mutually agree that although this headache is still a mystery it's obviously bothering her a lot. The painkillers are working so are continued, and Doctor B promises to look up her symptoms in his reference books in time for her next appointment the following week. Jill leaves feeling a good deal better than she had an hour before.

Consultation styles and outcomes

This simple analogy hopefully illustrates some fundamental differences in the style of the two consultations, but also several similarities.

Neither doctor had any idea what was causing Jill's headaches, but this was a problem only for Doctor A, who finds it hard to deal with conditions that he can't understand or name. He tends to think these are not serious conditions. Doctor B was much better at recognising the fact that, whatever was going on, it was causing significant difficulties, which therefore made it a serious problem. Doctor B was open about his puzzlement over the cause of the symptoms and wanted to look into it further. Doctor A preferred to keep it to himself when he was unsure of a problem and only wanted to look into it further if Jill persisted in complaining of the symptoms.

Both doctors actually hated running behind time in their surgeries but whereas Doctor A would take steps to bring a consultation to a close if it looked like going on for a while, Doctor B would go with the flow, and go on a bit longer. Often this irritated the next patient if they didn't know him well enough, but once they realised he always ran a bit behind time they would just show up a bit later for their appointment or bring a book to read.

Both Doctor A and Doctor B are good doctors. Looking at their prescribing habits or clinical skills in handling conditions like asthma or diabetes will probably not show any differences, and certainly Doctor A is well liked and respected by his patients. A more detailed analysis of the sorts of patients and problems that the two doctors deal with best shows, however, that Doctor A is not so good at handling the more ill-defined illnesses that are very commonly seen in general practice, or those that get the label of 'psychological illness'. The commonest way he deals with this is to attach recognised 'physical' diagnoses to everything he can. So in the case of Jill, had he seen her again it would be quite likely that he'd call these headaches 'a sort of migraine', which would justify his prescribing anti-migraine treatment for a while. This would not work, as these are not migraine headaches, and ultimately Doctor A would admit that he couldn't help Jill (although not in so many words) and that he'd like her to see a neurologist about the headaches. Should that prove unhelpful his back-up plan is to refer Jill to a psychologist.

Doctor B would be unlikely to prescribe anti-migraine treatment because he'd recognise these were not migraines Jill was describing. In fact, he couldn't really work out what was causing the headaches, but in the course of the next several consultations he'd gather much more information about what Jill was like as a person and how her condition was affecting her life. He might well also refer Jill to a neurologist and a psychologist during the course of trying to help her but he would do so within the context of treating Jill, and not with the hope of passing the buck to another doctor or therapist, as was really the case with Doctor A.

The preceding scenario could of course just as easily have been about CFS/ME as about headaches. It is very likely that the contrast between the two doctors would have been even more striking if it had been. Doctor A has pretty fixed views about CFS/ME, having seen quite a few patients with it over the preceding years. Like a lot of doctors who work in the same way as him, he calls CFS/ME a 'heartsink' condition, meaning that his heart sinks when another patient comes in complaining of 'feeling tired all the time'. In doing so he wrongly puts everyone with fatigue in the one diagnostic basket because he doesn't recognise CFS/ME as a condition in its own right. If you could get him to admit what he really thinks about people with CFS/ME or any sort of fatigue you'd find he doesn't have a high opinion of them. He has a superior attitude to people who 'buckle under stress' because, as a doctor, he has to cope with a high and stressful workload every day. So when someone comes in saying, 'You know, doctor I feel tired all the time', he has to suppress the desire to reply with, 'So do I, but I have to get on with life. Now, what's your problem?'

Doctor B is, if anything, under more stress than Doctor A because over the years he has accumulated a large number of patients who recognise that he is good at dealing with conditions that have a psychological component. Dealing with the more fundamental aspects of what makes people tick is more time consuming and draining of him personally than the consultation style of his colleague. He's a good listener and while not shy of using modern medicines carefully he is also willing to explore complementary therapies (which Doctor A dismisses as quackery).

The essential difference between the two doctors is that Doctor A needs a diagnosis before he can do anything else whereas Doctor B only needs an ill patient in order to start working. As a consequence of his mindset Doctor A sees physical and psychological illnesses as distinct and needing separate attention but Doctor B makes no distinction and always moves on both fronts.

Doctor A's black and white view of 'fatigue' obscures the detail of the different conditions that can cause it. He is quite likely to be able to diagnose depression and anxiety states efficiently because these are established in the medical literature and there are diagnostic tools such as questionnaires that can help him make those diagnoses (although as we've previously seen these are only aids to the recognition of patterns of behaviour). Modern antidepressant treatment is effective so even if he is not as good as Doctor B at getting in tune with the psyche of his patients he isn't completely ineffective at dealing with mood disorders in general. But he is heavily reliant on drug therapy to achieve his results and for many patients this is either unsatisfactory or incomplete or both. He's particularly stuck if his patients don't respond to prescription medicines and then he relies on other professionals, such as psychologists to take over completely. As the availability of psychological therapy within the NHS is very much less than is justified by the need this can leave his patients suspended without much in the way of help for months unless they go for private treatment.

Doctor B's acceptance that he can't diagnose everything and that he can treat from the start without fully understanding the exact nature of the illness makes it possible for him to help people with complex problems including CFS/ME. He is non-judgemental in assessing someone's character and doesn't lump people together under simple headings.

There is nothing new in this approach and in fact all good doctors used to work this way. Only within the past 150 years has science begun to 'explain' the biology of health and illness. Prior to the modern era only a few truly effective remedies were known and the practice of medicine was principally a skill based on an understanding of human behaviour and the need for wise advice. Discovering that this is still the basic level at which the relationship between the ill person and the doctor needs to work can come as a revelation to some modern doctors, who are over-trained to be scientists first. Achieving this shift in attitude and translating it into how a doctor practises medicine within the constraints of the present health services is, however, no easy task.

Real life medicine

Doctor A and Doctor B do exist, but not often in the clearly contrasting forms just presented. Like their patients, doctors are also human, complex and different. The great majority of doctors share some of the qualities of both Doctor A and Doctor B and in fact may oscillate between different consulting styles according to their own mood, the amount of time available or other influences particular to the individual consultation.

DOCTOR VARIABILITY

The pressures on all health professionals are now greater than they have ever been. Much more is now known about many important common diseases and ensuring that guidelines of good management are met for them is very time consuming. However, the structure of delivering care in general practice is fundamentally the same as it was when the NHS was established in 1948. The practice team has grown since those days to incorporate reception staff and typists, practice nurses, health visitors, community general and psychiatric nurses, midwives and more but the basic consultation format is a short meeting between one doctor and one patient and remains the same. Standards of medical training in Britain are high and the range of skills a British GP needs to have are considerable, but no doctor can excel in every field. In group practices there is a bit of scope for patients to 'shop around' until they find a doctor they feel they get on with but most people don't like to do this and feel a certain amount of allegiance to the first doctor they see. In many places there is little or no choice of doctor anyway.

Although there are some systems of review that can detect when a doctor is doing a particularly bad job they operate at only the crudest levels, and a doctor needs to be pretty incompetent to be noticed by the system. Although doctors do need to undertake periodic updates in their knowledge, modern medicine is so vast that it is impossible to keep up to date with more than a fraction of it. Within such a system it is inevitable that there will be a certain number of Doctor A look-alikes, which is bad news if you have CFS/ME and he (or she) is your GP.

One other important aspect of doctor variability that doesn't often get talked about in the public arena is the health status of those who deliver the care. Doctors themselves have higher than average levels of depression, suicide, alcoholism and marital difficulty than the average in the population. General practice in the UK is going through yet another period of uncertainty driven by a host of factors including workload and political involvement, and satisfaction with the job is lower now than it has ever been. Nurses also feel undervalued and are certainly underpaid. The mental health needs of health care professionals is a subject for another book but in brief one can say that it is a minefield and one that rarely gets adequate attention. People who are stressed themselves do not find it easy to deliver a good service to those who look to them for professional advice that involves an element of emotional support too. This is one of the main reasons that Doctor A is less than sympathetic to people with chronic fatigue – because he's privately aware that he's fatigued himself but feels trapped and overwhelmed by the job and is reluctant to discuss his own needs frankly with a colleague. Doctors tell their patients to discuss their worries and that it will help them to do so, but they are not good at taking their own advice.

TIME PRESSURE AND MANAGEMENT

But even when your GP is more of the Doctor B type there are several potential blocks that can get in the way of the consultation process. Time is the main enemy. The average time for a GP consultation in the UK is only eight minutes – hardly enough to cover a complex medical situation. Doctor B is willing to stretch the consultation time but there is a limit to how far he can do that and still keep a semblance of order to the working day. Few patients are happy to be kept waiting half an hour or more for their booked appointment when the patient before them is pouring their heart out to the doctor, even though they may well do exactly the same when it's their turn.

One of the advantages of the British system of general practice is that the doctor can repeatedly see the same patient, thus making it possible to deal with a problem over several sessions, but managing this aspect of the consultation can be tricky. No one wants a clock ticking on the wall that rings when your time's up and tells you to leave and let the next patient in. Many studies have shown that patients markedly underestimate how much time has gone by in a consultation and it would also be very inhibiting to feel that you had to rush through all that you wanted to say in just a few minutes. Time management of the consultation is therefore a skill that the doctor has to have and doing this sensitively, without taking too much control of the consultation in Doctor A fashion, can take many years of experience. Often a patient will indeed feel reluctant to say all that they want to say, knowing that 'doctors are busy' and so the real reason for the consultation may well remain unspoken. Then the doctor needs to be able to pick up the cues in body language that tell him or her that the patient needs more time to get to the issues that are really bothering them. On a busy Friday evening surgery with a packed waiting room it's sometimes going to happen that this opportunity will be missed, or sidestepped.

The CFS/ME experience

It's easy to see that someone with CFS/ME can fall foul of an overstretched medical system. It has been a controversial condition for years, and many medical sceptics still remain who doubt its validity. The Chief Medical Officer's report won't convert these doctors overnight and certainly won't provide more hours in the day for them to do a better job of helping their patients. People with CFS/ME are, to those doctors who believe they know enough about the science of health and illness, physically healthy. People with CFS/ME feel bemused and let down if not taken seriously.

Those doctors who do try to address their patient's distress properly don't find themselves well supported in terms of specialists in CFS/ME who can offer extra advice. Ancillary services such as clinical psychology, which can be helpful for some people, are woefully lacking. However, there is a way through this presently unsatisfactory situation. In fact, some people with CFS/ME who have had excellent support from their doctor and other health care professionals might well be reading this and wondering what the fuss is about. It's impossible to quantify what proportion of people with CFS/ME do find themselves poorly served by the medical services compared to those who do not – one tends to hear more about the bad experiences than the good.

The route through CFS/ME for the sufferer depends on having good information about the condition, and hopefully the contents of this book will fill any gaps in knowledge. In the last part of the book we'll cover the types of treatment available. The next points are about getting the best from the medical system as it presently exists, imperfect as it may be.

Helping the system to work for you

1. BOOK ENOUGH TIME

When booking the appointment – especially your first appointment, when the doctor has got the most to do to get a feel for what is going wrong – ask for a double appointment. Quite simply the receptionist puts two appointments back to back. Most if not all practices do this when necessary and when it is known in advance that the standard appointment is going to be too short. Most practices book appointments at either seven and a half or ten-minute intervals. The former is certainly too short for any detailed assessment of a person's emotional well-being, and ten minutes is not much better. Two appointments allow 15 or 20 minutes, which is a much more comfortable time slot. It still won't be enough to cover everything, but a good start can be made. If you can't get a double appointment (and even if you can) then expect to get only part way through your assessment of what's wrong the first time you meet the doctor. Saying that you realise this at the start of the consultation defuses the time pressure.

2. WRITE DOWN YOUR SYMPTOMS

It doesn't need to be a work of literature – just a few notes will do. Not only will it remind you what to mention, but it can prove very helpful to the doctor. Perhaps, if you've gone into great detail, the doctor will need to read some of it after the appointment, but do it if you can.

3. LEAVE YOUR INTERNET PRINT-OUTS AT HOME!

If you have already looked into CFS/ME and accumulated a lot of information about it, don't bring it with you to the consultation. Although a good doctor wants his or her patients to be well informed they don't have the time in a surgery setting to judge the quality of what you have been reading. You can come back to the issue of reliable information about CFS/ME. Of course this issue goes both ways – your doctor may be the one with the knowledge gap. There is so much information around that it is impossible for a busy doctor to keep current in every topic. He may well be unaware of the Chief Medical Officer's report, for example, and be glad to know about it.

4. REMEMBER THAT SEVERAL APPOINTMENTS MAY BE REQUIRED

It is unlikely that even the most clued-up doctor will make a confident diagnosis of CFS/ME the first time he meets a new patient. The conditions that need to be remembered that can overlap with CFS/ME were covered in chapter 2 and it is very reasonable that the doctor should wish to check the basic laboratory investigations that were mentioned there too (blood and urine tests). These can take a week or so to come back, during which time the doctor can reflect on any extra information you might have provided, such as your summary of your symptoms. Quite often several shorter appointments actually achieve more than one or two long ones, as there is time between meetings to reflect on the issues and to read up relevant information.

5. REMEMBER THAT YOU ARE THE ONLY PERSON WHO KNOWS HOW YOU FEEL

You are unwell when you say so, not when you've had a diagnostic label applied. So you don't need to make excuses for feeling unwell. CFS/ME is real condition, not the absence of something else for which doctors have a test. Hopefully this is not territory that you'll be getting into if your doctor is well informed and a good listener. If you are unlucky enough to get a sceptical response from your GP concerning CFS/ME then you need point 6.

6. IF THERE SEEMS TO BE A COMMUNICATION ISSUE, DISCUSS IT

Even Doctor A would be put out if he really thought that his approach and reaction to his patient with CFS/ME was causing hurt or offence. Despite their prejudices, and even their private jibes about heartsink patients, very few doctors wish to be other than helpful. So if you sense that you are not being listened to or have some other grievance about the doctor's response then just say so! It needn't be put as a complaint, but as a statement of how you feel about the experience of being a patient at that time. For example, you could ask the doctor what his or her own views are concerning CFS/ME (assuming you've got to the stage that this is the likely diagnosis or seems so to you). If there seem to be entrenched views on the other side then at least you'll know that it is unlikely to be worth your while pursuing your case with this particular doctor. Such confrontations can become nasty and unpleasant for both parties and will be pretty certain to make you feel worse. Rather than getting to that stage it would be best to seek another opinion early on.

7. SEEING ANOTHER DOCTOR

If you are unhappy with some aspect of the way your doctor is treating you and this can't be resolved by discussion, or if you don't feel you want to discuss it, then you are perfectly entitled to seek another opinion. Within a group general practice you need do no more than make an appointment with another partner in the group. Should there be another surgery in your area then you just need to register with them. You don't need to give any explanation or ask anyone's say so. A practice will decline to take on new patients only in exceptional circumstances such as in those parts of the country where there are problems recruiting more GPs and therefore list sizes are already very high.

Such drastic change as re-registering is not something that most people wish to undertake and for many people outside the conurbations the option of another nearby surgery to register with does not exist. A second opinion from a specialist doctor should, however, pose no difficulty for your GP to arrange. If a doctor is confident of his or her own management of a patient then they will be only too happy to have their views confirmed by a colleague, whereas if they are unsure of what is wrong with a patient, or what best to do about their condition then they should be seeking another opinion anyway. So asking for a second opinion is not going to cause offence. The difficulty with CFS/ME is that very few doctors have developed a special interest in the condition, so there aren't many specific clinics around. As a result, patients are often seen by specialists in vaguely related medical disciplines such as rheumatology. That need not be a bad idea as many of the principles of treating any sort of persistent disability are common to all illnesses but the waiting time for an appointment is still likely to be long. The most controversy arises when the doctor is the one suggesting a second opinion – from a psychiatrist or psychologist.

8. PSYCHIATRY AND PSYCHOLOGY
Psychiatrists are medical doctors who have undergone specialist further training in the management of mental illness. Psychologists are not

usually doctors but are experts in human behaviour. There is a degree of overlap between these disciplines and they commonly work in concert. Mental illness, in all its forms, is the commonest ailment that affects human beings so it defies logic that there still tends to be a negative view of psychiatric and/or psychological illness in the general population. As we stated earlier, there has to be a psychological component to any illness and at times it is the dominant one. Although Doctor A might use a referral to one of these types of health professional because he can't think of anything better to do, the Doctor Bs of this world would take a more holistic view. If there isn't a formal psychiatric illness present, then a psychiatrist is only going to confirm that. A psychologist can usually offer helpful advice on coping with any illness, so either way one has nothing to lose and perhaps a lot to gain by seeing one of these individuals in the course of assessing or treating CFS/ME. The important point is to approach such a referral with a positive view, and not as an indication that you aren't being taken seriously.

9. THERE IS NO MAGIC BULLET FOR CFS/ME

Instead there are several different treatment options and it may take some experimentation to get the right mix for you. During this time there will probably be some setbacks. By definition CFS/ME lasts for months, so it is not a quick-fix illness. Pacing your expectations from the start will help you cope with the time scale, but this is admittedly a lot easier to say than to do.

10. MOST PEOPLE GET BETTER EVENTUALLY

A proportion of people with CFS/ME have a protracted illness that goes on for many years. The ME Association estimates that 25 per cent of people get the 'severe' type of illness, which makes them house, wheelchair or bed-bound. Insufficient research has been done into

CFS/ME to predict with any reliability what will be the course of the condition in an individual. Most people do improve in time, although they may remain prone to relapse at a future date. When the illness comes on suddenly, say after an acute virus infection, then it tends to have a better long-term course than when it comes on gradually. The longer the symptoms are present, the longer they are likely to remain that way. Co-existent mental health problems can prolong CFS/ME, emphasising the need to recognise and address them.

Working together

If the foregoing has suggested that everyone with CFS/ME has a battle to be taken seriously by health professionals then that was not the intention. Some people have had bad experiences, but fewer do so now and fewer still will do so in the future. The relationship between a person and his or her doctor is a valuable one based on mutual respect but when things do go wrong they can usually be sorted out by discussion. Despite real difficulties in manpower and resource availability within the modern NHS the overwhelming majority of health professionals manage to provide a decent, even excellent service and certainly all want to. Once the diagnosis of CFS/ME has been confirmed then both doctor and patient have to be prepared for the long haul. We don't yet have enough understanding of this illness and the simple acceptance of that fact should be enough to get people out of their trenches and into co-operating to tackle it.

Chapter 5

Treatments for CFS/ME

Evidence-based medicine

Over the past decade there has been a strong drive to critically appraise the ways in which every aspect of medical practice is carried out in a more rigorous fashion than used to be the case. This applies to methods of diagnosis, categorisation of illness, treatments, follow-up, the value of screening and so on. It has been given the general name of 'evidence-based medicine', which obviously implies that there is some other type of medicine that is not evidence-based. If it is a surprise to the public to know that some of the methods and treatments used by doctors have little or no good evidence in their favour then they are not alone – it has been news to a lot of doctors too. Many of the things that get done in medicine are done for no better reason than that they have always been done that way, and it makes good sense to re-visit these ways of working, keeping the good ones and improving the others.

It's also necessary to keep the value of evidence-based medicine in perspective. It is impossible to apply its principles to every aspect of human health and for many conditions we don't yet have enough information to categorically say which is the best way to diagnose, treat or explain it. That is where we are with CFS/ME but enthusiasts for evidence-based medicine can forget this when looking at the available medical literature. Compared to conditions like asthma or diabetes the amount of research done into the treatment of CFS/ME is small but it is not insignificant – there are thousands of research papers on CFS/ME. However, some of it does not stand up well under critical appraisal, because the studies have been too small or over too short a time scale or have some other methodological fault. 'Scientist doctors' can certainly point to the 'evidence base' for CFS/ME as it presently exists and say that it is deficient. That's true, but equally true is the disability of the hundreds of thousands of people with CFS/ME so we have to interpret with care the knowledge we have and turn it into sensible advice.

What follows here are summaries of the different treatments that have been tried, along with an indication of the strength of evidence for or against their effect. It is possible that bigger studies of a presently dubious treatment will reveal that it does work, and the opposite is also true.

Before describing the treatments, it is important to consider two more general aspects of illness recovery.

RECOGNISING AND NAMING THE ILLNESS

The value of a positive diagnosis is very high. This is especially true when the diagnosis is of a benign or otherwise harmless condition. Every doctor knows how gratifying it can be to see a patient worried about a lump that on examination is confirmed as unimportant. The relief on the patient's face can be priceless. But even when the condition is CFS/ME, which isn't fatal but can hardly be said to be harmless, the knowledge that it is not something like cancer or a degenerative nerve disease is a boost in itself. This is a point that needs to be remembered most by the 'scientist doctors', who think CFS/ME is an imaginary condition, or that it is a 'psychological' illness as though that in itself were enough explanation.

DEFINING THE AIMS OF TREATMENT

The ideal treatment for any illness removes the abnormal condition, replaces it with full health and removes the risk of the illness recurring. On such criteria medicine is almost entirely ineffectual – there are very few true cures. Realistically, treatment is therefore about moving towards a state of improved health and towards the reduction of symptoms and disability. The best treatment of any illness might only go part of the way down each of these tracks. There is no therapy for CFS/ME that will make it go away, so the goal of treatment has to be the maximum improvement of well-being and not the elimination of the primary condition, much as we all hope for that to become possible some day.

General categories of treatment

A detailed technical report on CFS/ME treatments was published by the National Health Service Centre for Reviews and Dissemination at the University of York in September 2002. It is available on line at http://www.york.ac.uk/inst/crd/report22.pdf, but be warned: it is nearly 130 pages long.

Treatments can be grouped under several general headings:

- Behavioural
  - ○ Cognitive behaviour therapy
  - ○ Graded exercise and pacing

- Immune system
- Drug therapies
  - Antiviral
  - Antidepressants
  - Sleep promotion (hypnotics)
  - Steroids and other hormones
- Dietary supplements
- Complementary medicine

Behavioural

The basic principle underlying behavioural treatments states that being ill can be prolonged by wrongly held beliefs concerning the illness, and that modifying these beliefs and the behaviour that stems from them will make a person feel better.

COGNITIVE BEHAVIOURAL THERAPY

The primary type of treatment is called 'cognitive behavioural therapy', or CBT, and a few studies have shown it to be an effective way to achieve improvement in CFS/ME, at least for some people. However, CBT has had a mixed reception from some experts and many patients, for several reasons.

If CBT is taken to imply that CFS/ME is 'just psychological' or 'all in the mind' then of course it would deserve to be treated with contempt. If one drops that idea but instead accepts the more helpful view that human behaviour is extremely diverse then it makes sense that when ill it is possible to get into a frame of mind that can amplify or create problems. Taking a simple example from earlier in the book, anxiety over a harmless lump causes all the feelings of stress until the doctor confirms that we have nothing to worry about. We didn't ask for the lump to appear but our belief that the lump might be cancerous generated a temporary illness of its own. Similarly no one asks to get

CFS/ME, but worry over what it might mean to be so dramatically unwell when previously healthy will undoubtedly cause alarm until a positive diagnosis is made. The problem with CFS/ME of course is that it does not go away once it's been given a name. In the case of the lump we can choose to ignore it if it's too small to bother about, or have it removed surgically if it's a nuisance, but these are options that we can decide about at our leisure because the worry has been removed. What the proponents of CBT in relation to CFS/ME are saying is that the persistence of illness changes our behaviour in a way that can amplify the symptoms or even create new ones. Anyone who has had a bad bout of the flu knows that they are 'not themselves' for a few days and the behaviour theory in chronic illness is this on a larger scale. Behaviour therapists do not say that they can explain why CFS/ME starts in the first place, only that they have a system of tackling its effects.

The main difficulty with CBT is that it generally needs to be carried out in conjunction with a therapist. Between 10 and 20 one-hour sessions would be the norm, with 'homework' to be done between sessions. This of course is a major stumbling block, because the number of suitably trained therapists (usually psychologists) working within the NHS is small and waiting times of over a year are not uncommon. In some parts of the UK clinical psychology is virtually non-existent, consequently many people seek private treatment. Provided it is approached in a positive way CBT will not make anyone worse, but it won't always help either. It can't be reliably predicted who will and won't benefit.

Other ways of delivering CBT, such as in the form of interactive computer programs, exist for some medical conditions but not yet for CFS/ME.

GRADED EXERCISE

Some confusion exists about what exactly is meant by this. It is clear that many people with CFS/ME who try to keep going at their old, pre-illness pace, or who push themselves hard in an effort to force recovery, can cause themselves more harm than good in the short term as they are likely to activate more symptoms. Similarly it is too simple to say that someone with CFS/ME, who has become very sedentary and therefore has become unfit, needs to get fitter to get better. Re-training the body to cope with more effort is a two-edged sword and needs to be approached with care and common sense. Graded exercise is therefore *not* the same as the 'pull up your socks and get on with it' type of advice that is insulting to patients and doesn't work anyway. Furthermore, graded exercise has to be sensitive to the individual's particular circumstances – it is generally not helpful to give the same programme of steadily increasing activity to everyone.

Two or three of the reasonably large trials done in graded exercise showed benefit. The ways in which the trials were conducted were based on set increases in exercise over several weeks rather than a totally flexible system of pacing and some of the studies had quite high drop-out rates. On balance graded exercise is a valid form of treatment for some people.

PACING

Pacing means living within a given envelope of activity defined on the basis of how much someone can do comfortably. By managing their energies conservatively they can therefore extend their periods of activity. Rest periods are important and with the passage of time one should see improvement. Pacing makes a lot of sense yet seems to have drawn criticism from some experts, who feel it can reinforce patterns of ill health or discourage rehabilitation. Surely this need not be so. Very few people with CFS/ME can be keen to keep feeling unwell and the vast majority are looking for treatment or at least support on the way out of the illness. If pacing is taken to mean permanent advice never to exceed a certain level of activity defined at the start of the illness then the criticism is justified – the concept of eventual improvement is essential to motivate and encourage someone, especially during the bad spells. But bad spells do occur and a sensible approach to rest, recuperation and moving on again positively makes good sense.

DISORDERED SENSE OF EFFORT
An interesting aside here, which is really to do with the cause of CFS/ME, is a concept proposed by workers looking at the effect of exercise and rehabilitation programmes in the condition. In one study people with CFS/ME were significantly weaker than the comparison groups and had the sensation of a high degree of effort at levels of muscular activity that were relatively low compared to people without CFS/ME. This suggests the possibility that in CFS/ME there is an abnormality of the sense of effort, so that people feel much more easily fatigued despite having apparently normal muscles. If correct this would explain the discrepancy between the lack of abnormalities on presently available tests and the marked sense of fatigue usually experienced in CFS/ME.

Immune system

As subtle abnormalities of the immune system have been proposed as possible causes of CFS/ME several types of treatment have been tried that one way or another have immune system effects. The results have been disappointing, although not entirely negative. Injection of antibody protein (immunoglobulin G, IgG) was tested in several trials, some of which showed partial benefit, others showed none and all had significant side effects from the treatment. As immunoglobulin is prepared from donated blood there is a small risk of transmission of infection from it.

Ampligen is an expensive drug still under evaluation in CFS/ME but in the one published trial so far it showed benefit and was well tolerated. It is not available in the UK and there is insufficient information to recommend it.

Drug therapies

ANTIVIRAL

The logic behind using antiviral treatment stems from the possible role of virus infection in causing CFS/ME. Interferon is a protein produced naturally by the body during viral infections and which has antiviral and immune system actions. It can now be manufactured artificially and has several uses in medicine such as in the treatment of hepatitis B and C virus infections. Two studies of interferon in CFS/ME reported some improvement, but not in all those treated. The antiviral drug aciclovir is not effective in CFS/ME.

ANTIDEPRESSANTS

There are several reasons why it can be worthwhile to use an antidepressant in CFS/ME. Several symptoms of depression, such as fatigue and sleep disturbance, are also found in CFS/ME and it is theoretically likely that there are some similarities in the brain chemistry changes underlying both conditions. The overlap is probably small as only a small proportion of people with CFS/ME benefit from antidepressants unless they also have other symptoms of a depressive illness. As with depressive illness any benefit could take several weeks to materialise but if there is no effect at about six weeks then there is little point in persevering.

There are several groups of antidepressant drug, the most commonly prescribed now being those related to Prozac (fluoxetine), which was the first of the 'selective serotonin re-uptake inhibitor' class, or SSRI for short. The earlier class of antidepressants, called the tricyclics, are still in wide use and tend to be more sedative than the SSRIs. As sleep disturbance is a common feature of CFS/ME then using a small dose of a tricyclic antidepressant (such as dothiepin or amitriptyline) helps some people with CFS/ME to sleep. Conversely the sedation of tricyclics might be too much for some people or could increase fatigue, so there are pros and cons. An untested hypothesis concerning the possible brain chemistry origins of CFS/ME has suggested the use of a group of antidepressants called the monoamine oxidase inhibitors (MAOIs). Although not outmoded, these drugs date from the early days of antidepressant research and are used only rarely now. In the one trial that looked at an MAOI called phenelzine there was, however, no improvement over six weeks of use.

Reluctance to take antidepressants can stem from several reasons. Media scares about their safety have done a disservice to these medicines, particularly the SSRIs, which are among the safest of all prescription drugs. Perhaps stronger is the stigma that attaches to all 'mental illness' in our society. So long as there is a view that depression is a second-class illness then antidepressants will be tarred with the same brush. Critics of using antidepressants in CFS/ME need to be sure that they are not actually voicing a prejudice in disguise. This does not mean that antidepressants are a panacea for CFS/ME (they are not), should be prescribed for everyone (this is an individual decision), have a strong research base for their use (it is weak) or that CFS/ME is a psychiatric illness (we've already dismantled that argument). It just means that they help some people and in the absence of a test to detect who they might be then a trial period of treatment is a sensible option to discuss.

As with any chronic illness, depression can result from the restrictions imposed by being ill. One therefore needs also to be alert to the fact that someone with CFS/ME can become depressed somewhere down the line and this needs to be noticed. Leaving depression untreated is a sure way of prolonging a person's ill health.

SLEEP PROMOTION

Sleep deprivation is an effective form of torture and conditions or circumstances associated with disruption to sleep are invariably associated with fatigue. Although a great deal of information is now known about the changes within the body and the brain that occur during sleep we have only a patchy idea of why sleep is so important. A simple explanation is that during sleep the electrical and chemical functions of the brain and nervous system are reset and recalibrated ready for the next wave of wakefulness and the levels of messenger chemicals within the system are replenished. A technological analogy is of a sophisticated computer system updating its data and clearing the clutter out of its memory to allow space for the barrage of information we take in constantly when awake.

Very little research has been done into the relationship between sleep disturbance and CFS/ME but more information could potentially be very helpful if the knowledge gained in depression is any guide. Rapid eye movement (REM) sleep is the phase of sleep when dreaming occurs and is named thus because in this stage the person's eyes flick rapidly around under their closed eyelids. During REM sleep our brain is very active and, other than the eye muscles, our main muscles are effectively paralysed. We go through several cycles of REM sleep each night, each one preceded by deepening levels of sleep which then reverses as REM sleep is in fact quite light – we are nearly awake during it. In depression there are decreased amounts of deep sleep and increased amounts of REM sleep in the early part of the night. Also, the time taken for the first episode of REM sleep to occur is reduced in depression – this pattern can sometimes persist in someone who has recovered from depression but who goes on to have another episode of it.

Clearly these observations are telling us something about the chemistry of the brain even if we do not fully understand what it is. The fact that we are almost paralysed during REM sleep (although we can regain muscle power instantly on waking) throws up an interesting potential link with the theory mentioned earlier that in CFS/ME there could be a disordered sense of effort. Admittedly this is highly speculative but it is not impossible to see how in some way not yet discovered the profound fatigue experienced in CFS/ME relates to the same type of changes in brain function that paralyse us during REM sleep.

There is more to getting a good night's sleep than not being awake for a few hours, which is probably why medicines to make people sleep (hypnotics) can have disappointing results. The sleep thus gained is not necessarily refreshing – a point often remarked upon by people with CFS/ME. There is also the grogginess factor of still having some drug in the system in the morning. Most of all there are the problems of long-term dependence on hypnotics. If someone has a particularly difficult time getting to sleep without medication then taking a regular hypnotic is probably the lesser of two evils.

Further information on getting a consistently good night's sleep is in chapter 7.

STEROIDS AND OTHER HORMONES

There are many naturally occurring hormones in the body that collectively come under the heading of 'steroids'. Usually the term refers to those hormones produced by the adrenal glands – two walnut-sized pieces of highly specialised tissue that are situated at the top of each kidney. The steroids produced here have very important roles in controlling salt and water balance, blood pressure and general metabolism. Failure of steroid production by the adrenal glands gives rise to a rare condition in which fatigue is prominent. The adrenal glands are controlled by other hormones arising in the pituitary gland of the brain, and it was mentioned in chapter 3 that some evidence exists that points to abnormalities in pituitary gland function as being a cause of CFS/ME. Significant steroid deficiencies have not been found, however, nor have trials of steroid drugs been shown to be significantly beneficial. In one small trial a short-lived improvement was seen in fatigue levels. Trials using higher doses of steroid gave no extra benefit but produced more side effects.

Sex hormones are also steroids, produced by the ovaries or testes. Again no evidence exists to tie changes in sex steroid levels to CFS/ME. Some women with CFS/ME may experience a change in the level of symptoms during the course of their menstrual cycle or during pregnancy. Changing sex hormone levels, for example with hormone replacement therapy, does not help.

Dietary and vitamin supplements

In one trial comparing injections of magnesium with placebo (dummy treatment) over six weeks the treatment group had a significantly better outcome. In another study levels of magnesium within the red cells of the blood were low in CFS/ME, but other studies have not confirmed this. Evening primrose oil has produced conflicting results, with one study reporting benefit after three months of taking 4 grams daily and another, using the same dose, showing no benefit.

Vitamin B12 is essential for the manufacture of red blood cells and the maintenance of the 'insulating' material that covers nerve tissue (myelin). It is absorbed from foods of animal origin in the presence of a substance called intrinsic factor, normally made by cells in the stomach lining. Intrinsic factor binds to vitamin B12 first in the stomach and the combination is then absorbed downstream in the small bowel. Vitamin B12 is stored in the liver; at any one time we have about three years' supply there. In the condition called pernicious anaemia there is a failure of the stomach cells to produce intrinsic factor and ultimately a deficiency of vitamin B12 occurs. Some other conditions of the digestive system will also cause failure of vitamin B12 absorption, as would a strictly vegan diet over a long enough period of time. However, detectable vitamin B12 deficiency is uncommon and is usually hinted at by ordinary blood tests and easily confirmed by measuring the amount of the vitamin in the blood.

In contrast to the infrequency with which B12 deficiency is proven, vitamin B12 has long been used as a 'treatment' for fatigue and as an energy booster, both in human and in veterinary medicine. It undoubt-edly has a strong placebo effect (the response one gets from an inactive treatment if the person receiving it believes strongly enough that it works). Although vitamin B12 is an active substance, once the body's stores are topped up any excess is simply excreted in the urine, so there is no logic to using it outside of deficiency states. Vitamin B12 has been used in CFS/ME but not in trials sufficiently well designed to separate the real from the placebo effects. Anecdotal evidence suggests it can be helpful in about a third of patients.

NADH (nicotinamide adenine dinucleotide) is a substance that facilitates the energy-releasing reactions that occur within cells. In a small trial (33 patients) with CFS/ME, of those who took an oral supplement of NADH a small number had a modest improvement. A larger trial of this treatment is planned.

Carnitine and Co-enzyme Q10 (ubiquinone) are both 'energy-providing substances' that can be obtained from health food stores. There are no good trials of their use in CFS/ME but there is anecdotal support for their use in general fatigue.

Complementary medicine

To touch upon the use of complementary treatments, irrespective of the condition for which they are used, is to open up one of the widest fields of debate in medicine. There are plenty of contrasting, even opposite, views around within the public and especially the pro-fessional arenas. There are the devotees of evidence-based medicine who can't find the studies that show these therapies work better than placebo. There are also the many millions of satisfied users of complementary treatments who rightly have a better opinion of themselves than as simply gullible consumers or the victims of faddism.

In contrast to the vast resources of the conventional pharmaceutical industry, which spends billions of pounds annually on drug research, the amount of funding that goes into complementary research is tiny. There is little or no money to be made, in drug industry terms, in finding out if a particular type of herb is useful in treating CFS/ME because the treatment could not be patented or commercialised. If a condition is complex or difficult to assess and in particular if there is no 'test' for it then it becomes very much harder to study. Think of the differences in this respect between high blood pressure (easily measured with a desk-top instrument) and CFS/ME and you have a good idea why there should be orders of magnitude of difference in the amount of research work done in these conditions.

Of course, once you know a bit more about high blood pressure you find that the treatments that would have the most impact on the condition in the greatest number of people have nothing to do with which drug to choose, but instead are about changes in lifestyle and diet that we could all undertake. These are somewhat less attractive to the drug industry and are also much more difficult to implement, especially in the time-pressured environment of modern medical practice. Hence our present position.

Certainly there is a large body of medical literature on complementary treatments but it will never be comparable, either in quality or quantity, to that on 'conventional' treatments. For some doctors, and patients, that means that complementary medicine is a no-go area. For others who are willing to live with the fact that life isn't perfect then there is much to be gained from them.

Arguments over which treatment is better than any other are unhelpful because different conditions lend themselves to being treated in different ways. How to choose a suitable complementary therapy is outside the remit of this book. Homeopathy has the advantage of being available within the NHS, albeit to a limited degree. In a few areas NHS clinics in acupuncture and hypnotism are also available.

Complementary therapies tend to share a problem of sorts, which can happen in conventional medicine too, which is that it is difficult to separate the effect of the therapist from the effect of the treatment. Taking homeopathy as an example, a homeopathic consultation commonly lasts an hour, during which time the homeopath will take an extensive history of the symptoms and find out a lot of detail about what makes the patient's illness an individual one. Homeopaths, almost by definition, need to be good listeners and in itself this is therapeutic to someone who is ill, and who perhaps feels that they have not previously been listened to.

GPs would love to have the luxury of hour-long appointments. Not only would they find the practice of medicine less stressful, they would be better doctors for it. Sadly it's a pipe dream to do this for more than a fraction of the number of patients that a GP has to see. Many GPs have, however, undertaken some training in homeopathy or other forms of complementary medicine and try to use that within the limits of the surgery setting. Usually such a GP will volunteer this information or offer it spontaneously if he or she sees a patient for whom a complementary approach seems worthwhile. If not, then it is still worth asking what the doctor's views are of complementary treatments. They may be able to recommend known therapists and in some cases can refer you to an NHS service. Some complementary treatments are of dubious value even on the most generous analysis and many are very expensive, so at least make sure that you seek an accredited practitioner in the treatment. Appendix B lists contact information for some relevant organisations.

SUMMARY

- No single treatment stands out as the best for CFS/ME.
- The Chief Medical Officer's report listed cognitive behavioural therapy, graded exercise and pacing as the three most beneficial modes of treatment.
- There are significant limitations on the availability of these and other treatments in the UK.
- There is a small amount of supportive evidence for the use of immune system treatments, antidepressants, hypnotics, vitamin supplements, 'energy-boosters' and complementary therapies to help alleviate some of the symptoms of CFS/ME.

Chapter 6

A Treatment Scheme for CFS/ME

No one method of treatment stands out as better than any other and in the experience of this book's main author (DR) as a general practitioner a mixture of several approaches works better than one alone. The advice that now follows is a personal view that borrows both from published information on CFS/ME and from practical experience of treating patients with it.

One of the problems reported by many sufferers is the lack of specific guidance on how to tackle the condition and presented here is practical advice that the reader with CFS/ME will hopefully find helpful. Having stated earlier in the book that individual treatment is essential in CFS/ME it follows that it should be impossible to present a set scheme that will work for everyone. So although these points are perhaps the main ones you will need for dealing with CFS/ME, exactly how you do so will be up to you.

Some provisos are necessary. The first is that the diagnosis must be established by a qualified medical practitioner. This book is not about self-diagnosis and should not be used in such a way. Second, the role of your own medical adviser should remain central to the management of your illness. Although some doctors remain dismissive of CFS/ME and are therefore incapable of treating it, most are supportive and wish to be as helpful as possible. So long as your doctor's advice is working for you, then stick with it.

1. Accept the illness

The starting point of an illness is when you begin to feel unwell, not when the diagnosis has been made – ultimately someone will confirm that you have CFS/ME. As the onset can be abrupt and the amount of disability marked it can be a hard blow to accept this illness. In fact most people who get CFS/ME feel its onset is like a crash occurring in their life. Similarly those around them can feel bewildered and confused by what has happened so dramatically to a person previously quite well. Once you begin to learn more and find out that it can last for months or even years you can become very gloomy or properly depressed. CFS/ME is a disruptive illness, but it is not fatal. Most people recover and everyone can learn to live with it. It is possible to have a life and have CFS/ME and you need to focus your energies on doing so. We don't know why people get CFS/ME, but it happens every day. Ideas that some people with certain personality types are the only ones who are affected are wrong. Anyone can get CFS/ME. Such is the reality of the condition, though, that accepting the illness may be impossible until some recovery has already got underway.

2. Accept the equal importance of mind and body

This is the second part of accepting the illness. There is some evidence that patients who pursue a purely physical cause for CFS/ME may end up feeling ill for longer. Doctors who can't treat a condition until it has been 'scientifically proven' to exist aren't good at treating conditions like CFS/ME. Both positions may be driven partly by the desire to explain illness fully (which is a fair ideal but an impractical one) and partly by the mind/body split thinking that we've been taught to accept as standard. It's both healthier and more accurate to accept that being ill involves both physical and psychological components. By doing so you get rid of all the baggage that goes with so-called psychosomatic illness. Unless you act to improve both your mental and your physical well-being you will not make much progress with CFS/ME. (The same could probably be said of any illness.) So you need to accept that there will be work required in both areas.

3. Get connected

CFS/ME affects up to 200,000 people in the UK alone. Although having CFS/ME can be an isolating experience the truth is that someone near you has CFS/ME and is going through the same set of difficulties, or may be a lot further on the road to recovery. Their experiences can be invaluable to you in coming to terms with your own illness. The old saying that a problem shared is a problem halved has a lot of truth in it. You can make contact with other people with CFS/ME by looking for support groups or meetings in your local paper or phone book. The ME Association has recently expanded their support service (ME Connect), which is available by phone, fax or e-mail every day of the year (see appendix B). The Internet offers the chance to share experiences with people irrespective of their location. Care must be taken when using web-based discussion groups that you use one that is properly run, but good ones do exist. There is an active and helpful group on the NetDoctor web site at http://www.netdoctor.co.uk/discussion. (Properly organised boards allow you to set up an 'account' and a user name that lets you communicate with other users but does not display any personal information about you. Never post personal details such as your postal or e-mail address or telephone number on web groups.) The Internet allows you to be both frank and anonymous at the same time and can be a great source of support and encouragement.

4. Get a good doctor

We looked at this in chapter 4, so you could refresh your memory about this now. Unless you have no choice of local GP then you should seriously consider consulting another doctor if you can't get on with your present one and have been unable to resolve the difficulties by discussion. The ME Association has a database of doctors who have a special interest in CFS/ME so you could consider consulting one of them if you are at an impasse.

5. Get informed, be informative

Although this advice is now superfluous to you, other people you are in regular contact with need to be aware of the facts concerning CFS/ME. Having CFS/ME changes your life to a greater or lesser extent, and in doing so has an impact on those around you. It may influence your role and relationships at home, alter your working capacity, your working relationships and your social life. A lot of problems that arise from these changes are the result of inadequate or inaccurate information about CFS/ME. You don't want to wear a placard exclaiming you've got this illness but key people in your life need to be well informed. This book may assist in this regard and other information can be obtained from the ME Association. Ask your friends and colleagues to read it.

6. Map out your pre- and post-CFS/ME states

Another old saying goes something like 'you don't know what you've got until you've lost it'. When you were well, like most people, you didn't think much about what you'd get done in a day: how much distance you walked, how much time you spent on your feet, or at specific tasks at work, or cooking, reading or watching TV. When you have your energy sapped by CFS/ME then you soon notice all the things that you used to take for granted. Without getting into enormous detail you need to quantify what an ordinary day for you used to be like, because your ultimate aim is to get back to that level of activity. Go through a typical day in your mind's eye and write down an hour-by-hour account. Remember also to note how much sleep you used to get. Repeat the process for how you are now, noting particular factors that increase your symptoms. Some of the items on this list may be so problematic you will have to avoid them completely. For others you might be able to think of easier ways of doing the same task – splitting it up into shorter time scales for example or spreading a task over several days instead of cramming it all into one. For others, where you can put a figure against the amount of activity you used to do, then you can write down what level of activity represents 10 per cent of this, and 30 per cent, 50 per cent and so on up the scale. You can use this to guide your planning in the next steps.

7. Set priorities for improvement

What do you want to achieve first? For many this will mean getting back to paid employment, for others it will be to enjoy a pastime or sport and for some it will be managing to get out of the house for a walk. You'll actually want to do all of these things but if they are all given priority status then none of them will get done. It is not defeatist to accept that CFS/ME takes a while to recover from. If you set modest goals for improvement and exceed them then you will have good reason to be pleased. If you set unrealistic goals and fail to meet them you'll add insult to injury. Remember too though that *any improvement is a success in itself.*

Therefore, decide what you can drop and concentrate on the essentials. To get this off the ground try brainstorming a random list of what you want to do or achieve. Go down each of these ideas and then break them down further into their component parts. For example, you could put that getting back to work is your priority, but that is actually a complex task that needs to be broken down into the need to get up in the morning at the right time, dealing with transport services or driving, concentrating at work and so on.

Once you've rendered the big tasks down to their building blocks you can start to sort them further. It may help to do a sort of profit and loss analysis of these tasks. For each one give it a mark out of a hundred concerning its importance to you. Against it put a mark for the level of difficulty. For example, you might rate walking the dog every day as being 40 per cent important (profit) but 70 per cent difficult (loss) because it exhausts you. That's a 30 per cent loss so is not a feasible idea as it stands. On the other hand you might decide that walking the dog once a week drops the difficulty level because you give yourself time to recover (30 per cent this time). Now you are in profit so can think of taking it on. Decide on the amount of gain versus pain for each of the tasks listed and you'll soon have a list of realistic possibilities for your recovery plan.

8. Make a recovery plan

Having decided what your main aims are going to be, then decide how much time you will give yourself to make progress. You may need to take the advice of family, friends or your doctor at this point, as it's likely you'll want to go faster than might be feasible. Much depends on your present level of symptoms but at both ends of the scale of disability you should 'ca canny' as the Scots say.

If you are only mildly affected and coping with most daily activities or getting to work most days of the week and are managing financially then why push so hard that you risk upsetting this? If on the other hand you are pretty much housebound then for you small gains are large percentage improvements, so don't risk creating setbacks. Any progress is good progress and it is important to take heart from that. Frustration at 'slow' progress is perfectly understandable but is negative and erodes any gains you make. Where you may be in the most difficulty is if the CFS/ME persists long enough to cause secondary problems such as with employment. External pressures upon you to get better are much less under your control and may increase the stress of being ill.

9. Sort out employment issues

If you are in a job that protects your pay when off sick then it will be financially tolerable to be off work for a while, but you may perhaps be worried about the knock-on effects on later promotion. Few employers are as good as the best when it comes to dealing with ill employees. Ideally a phased recovery to work should be the norm but only a minority of employers manage to embrace this idea. Most require you to be fully fit to do a whole normal day's work or not be at work at all, and in some types of occupation no other option is possible.

Discuss if you can the possibility of coming back slowly by modifying your duties, being flexible about start and finish times, working part time for a bit or working from home. If you need to be off work completely then you will need to be signed off formally by your GP, and when that period of disability goes on for months you will find that the benefits system goes into action. Depending on the outcome of their deliberations you will be transferred to invalidity benefit if still unfit or will be told you are fit to work! Unfortunately the medical assessors cannot base their 'fitness to work' decision on whether someone is capable of returning to their old job, nor is it their role to provide someone with employment. This often gives rise to apparently unjust (and a fair few definitely unjust) decisions. The appeal process is lengthy and a common source of unnecessary stress to patients. Now that CFS/ME has been properly embraced by the Department of Health we might see less of this problem arising.

10. Sort out pain control

Painkillers may help muscle pains and it's best to start with the simple ones like paracetamol, using them at the correct dose and sufficiently often. Taking painkillers after a pain has come on is fine for occasional symptoms but if the pain is regular and you wait until you can't tolerate it before taking the medicine then you are always chasing along behind it and not getting full relief. Mixtures of paracetamol and codeine are slightly more effective but can cause constipation or nausea. Anti-inflammatory medicines of the ibuprofen family (called NSAIDs or non-steroidal anti-inflammatory drugs) are also worth trying but may cause indigestion and, rarely, allergic reactions. Aspirin has been noted to be more effective than some other analgesics, but again may cause stomach upset.

Many people with CFS/ME note that they get poor pain relief from conventional analgesics however there is some evidence that a low dose of tricyclic antidepressant such as amitriptyline can be an effective painkiller. At low doses one gets fewer of the side effects of these drugs, such as a dry mouth and constipation. This is particularly important as many people with CFS/ME are over sensitive to these drugs. Taking the dose in the evening may also help sleep, which is an important aspect of dealing with CFS/ME and is covered in the next chapter.

Acupuncture could be considered as a drug-free alternative, as could a TENS machine (transcutaneous nerve stimulator). This applies a tiny current through electrodes applied to the skin, which may block pain signals in the spinal cord. All of these treatments should be guided by your doctor.

11. Check out your illness beliefs and reactions

This is a bit like do-it-yourself cognitive behaviour therapy but it can be increased in value if you engage your partner or a friend or relative to work through it with you. The central reasoning in CBT is that our interpretation of symptoms of disease modifies our reactions to the disease in ways that can amplify or worsen the condition. By tackling these interpretations and steering them in a different direction we can positively influence our reactions to being unwell. Some examples will illustrate the point.

If, for the sake of argument, you strongly believe that your CFS/ME has a physical cause and cannot see yourself coping with the condition until that cause is identified and named then you will have a significant block to improvement for a long time to come. It might not be that you have formed this opinion in these exact terms. It may be instead that you are very frustrated to know that all your tests are normal when you know that there is something wrong with you. Here the illness belief is one of a need to identify the cause. The therapeutic response to this belief would run along the lines that you do not need to know the cause of an illness in order to begin healing from it. By accepting this belief you remove the block to improvement.

Often the 'two-column technique' is used to list original beliefs down one side and alternative, more helpful thoughts down the other. For example:

Original thought	**Alternative thought**
No one believes that I'm ill.	Hundreds of thousands of people, patients and doctors know that CFS/ME is a real illness
CFS is untreatable and lasts for years.	There are several treatment strategies that work. Some people are ill for years, others just for months. I can't tell in advance how long it will take me to get better.
If I get a relapse I'll be back to square one.	Relapses are common in CFS/ME. Improvement is a wavy line, not a straight one. I might get knocked back a bit, but not all the way.

Original thought	Alternative thought
I'll end up in a wheelchair.	This happens only to a very small minority of people with CFS/ME. Chance is on my side that I will not be so severely affected.
I've got to completely rest if I get tired or I'll get worse.	A balance between rest and activity is the best way to maintain my improvement.
I will lose my job.	CFS/ME is a valid reason to take time off work. I have been a good employee and I can keep working. I will find out about modifying my work patterns to let me cope.

To expand on these columns you can note your reactions to your illness as they occur. Ask yourself at the time what you think a symptom means and if you identify any negative associations with it. List alternative reactions (which is where it is helpful to have a partner) and focus on accepting these over the negative ones. Despite its simplicity this sort of technique can have a strong impact on the experience of illness.

12. Allow time for relaxation

Although the 'yuppie flu' label that was applied to CFS/ME a few years ago was quite wrong there is almost always some value in reassessing the stresses and strains that we put ourselves through on a daily basis, usually without much thought for the consequences. Particularly useful is deliberately making time for relaxation, and getting into the frame of mind that sees this as essential to overall well-being, and not a waste of time that could be better spent bombing around. There is a very wide range of ways in which you can do this. Yoga classes, meditation, massage and aromatherapy are popular for good reasons and they can encourage you to discover the lost art of relaxation. Perhaps you used to have a hobby that you enjoyed but which got sidelined by a lack of time, or there is some other pastime that you haven't previously tried but which takes your fancy. It need not be expensive – most of the investment is your time. Rest periods therefore need not be wasted time. Getting into the habit of making time for yourself should be a priority for everyone.

13. Consider complementary treatments

Discuss with your doctor whether a trial of NADH, carnitine, Co-enzyme Q10 or one of the other treatments listed in the previous chapter are worthwhile. Some of these are outside the normal range that a GP will use or have experience of, so it won't always be possible for the doctor to express an informed opinion on them. Hopefully most doctors have no objections to agreeing to safe treatments even if the chance of success is low.

Homeopathy is not a recipe-book type of treatment in which the diagnosis dictates the treatment, as so often is the case in conventional medicine. One can't therefore reliably suggest specific homeopathic remedies that will help in CFS/ME and the best option is to see a qualified homeopath. That should preferably be one who is also a doctor (anyone can call themselves a homeopath without any need for a qualification). Most pharmacies sell a range of 'low potency' homeopathic remedies straight to the public. Short of having a proper assessment these may be of most value in CFS/ME:

- Zincum metallicum
- Gelsemium
- Rhus toxicodendron.

14. Seek specialist advice

Where progress is very slow or the degree of disability very marked then specialist advice should be sought from a physician with a special interest in CFS/ME. It is very likely that your GP would wish to have a consultant's opinion in these circumstances anyway. Such specialists are very few in number so those in other medical specialties such as metabolic medicine (hormone abnormalities) or rheumatology (joint and soft tissue disease) are often those who see patients with CFS/ME. Only rarely will such a referral reveal some other diagnosis but it may lead to a line of treatment that has not already been tried and it is a route into rehabilitation services that are not directly available to your GP. Reassurance that everything possible is being done is valuable in itself.

Conversely, seeing a specialist in a different branch of medicine might lead to a diagnosis stemming from that consultant's own field of interest. Thus a rheumatologist might say (in good faith, but incorrectly) that you have fibromyalgia instead, or a heart specialist may label it as a slight heart problem called mitral valve prolapse. These are controversial conditions in their own right, and mixing them up with CFS/ME only magnifies the confusion surrounding the whole illness. Needless to say none of this helps the patients.

15. Maintain a positive outlook

Being chronically unwell can bring its own problems. Loss of self-esteem, financial hardship, fall in mood or increased anxiety over the future can all crowd in and at times perhaps make it look as if you will never get better. Contact with support organisations and with other people who have CFS/ME is invaluable when this happens, as is the support of your family and of your doctor. If real depression creeps in then it may need formal antidepressant treatment. You may find it almost impossible to improve without it. This is no admission of defeat, just an acknowledgement of the reality that CFS/ME is not an easy condition to cope with, no matter who you are.

Keep a long-term view of your condition – you can expect to get better in time and in the meantime you can learn to live within your limits. The power of positive feedback is strong, which is something for you to remember and for your friends and family to work at reinforcing. Ultimately you will shake it off and as time goes by better methods of treatment will arise. There's a much more positive attitude around now to CFS/ME and a lot of effort is going into tackling it properly after some years of neglect. That's very much to the good, and will benefit you sooner or later.

Chapter 7

Getting a Good Sleep

Sleeplessness is common in the general population. It can be caused by stress, pain, the need to pass urine, noisy neighbours, a partner who snores, having young children, an uncomfortable bed, shift work, some medicines, heavy or spicy food and drinks (e.g. alcohol and those containing caffeine, such as coffee and tea). CFS/ME is often accompanied by sleep disturbance but these other factors can just as easily coincide. Disturbed sleep can cause a great deal of distress and amplifies the symptoms of CFS/ME, so when present it needs effective treatment.

How much sleep is enough?

Everyone's needs are different. The range of time people sleep normally is as wide as three to ten hours. As a general rule of thumb, five to six hours' sleep is probably a minimum below which your intellectual performance will be affected but this need may be higher in CFS/ME. Most people need between seven and eight hours' sleep a night to feel refreshed. Generally, people require less sleep the older they get.

How to get a good sleep

Some general points may help you get back in the habit of sleeping well, which is very likely to have a positive effect on your condition. Not all of these tips might help, but hopefully some will.

- Establish a routine.
- Get up at the same time each morning, even if you have not had a good night's sleep. Don't sleep during the day, and don't go to bed early unless you are tired. You can't force yourself to sleep and going too soon will probably result in you just lying in bed thinking about problems.
- Take as much physical exercise during the day as safely makes you tired, bearing in mind the need to avoid overdoing it. Obviously this needs to be fitted in with your overall strategy for recovery.
- Avoid exercise for two hours before bedtime. This is because exercise 'activates' the body, which can make it difficult to get off to sleep.
- Avoid watching disturbing or violent films prior to bedtime.
- Avoid drinking caffeine (tea, coffee, cola) in the evening after 6 pm.
- Drink herbal teas or milky drinks such as Horlicks in the evening. Herbal teas don't contain caffeine and milky drinks are as good as sleeping tablets for many people. However, be aware that chocolate or cocoa-based milk drinks often contain caffeine.
- Avoid heavy meals two hours before bedtime. It can be difficult to get off to sleep with a full stomach.
- Avoid alcohol in the evening (many people with CFS/ME find they

need to avoid it completely). While alcohol is sedative, it is not a good idea to try to use it to sort out a sleep problem because it does not lead to normal restful sleep. In addition, alcohol stimulates the passage of urine, which further disrupts sleep.

- Associate your bedroom with sleep. Avoiding having a TV or radio there. The bedroom should be warm and familiar with a comfortable bed and quilt. Ideally, the room should be decorated in a relaxing way.
- Use aromatic oils in the bath or on your pillow, such as lavender, which can help relaxation.
- Use relaxation techniques, which you can learn from books or audiotapes. Reading in bed helps some people, but it can prevent others from getting off to sleep. If you do read in bed, only read light-hearted books or magazines.

If you are kept awake, or wake up worrying during the night, try the following:

- At least two hours before bedtime, write down the problems that keep you awake. Also write down the next step you need to take towards resolving each problem.
- If you find yourself thinking over the problems in bed, tell yourself you have the matter in hand and that going over it now will not help.
- If a new worry occurs during the night, write it down or commit it to memory and deal with it the next day.
- If you still do not manage to get to sleep, or you wake during the night and can't get back to sleep, get up. Do not lie in bed tossing and turning. Go and do something else like listening to relaxing music, having a warm bath or making yourself a milky drink. Go back to bed when you feel tired again.

If getting off to sleep becomes a preoccupation then:

- Do not try to fall asleep.
- Tell yourself that sleep will come and that relaxing in bed is nearly as good.
- Try to keep your eyes open. As they naturally try to close, tell yourself to resist for just another few seconds. This should tempt sleep to take over.
- If unhelpful thoughts pop into your mind, try and visualise a relaxing or pleasant scene.

Medicines to help sleep

Non drug-based methods to promote sleep are the first line but if insomnia persists there are several medications that can help.

BENZODIAZEPINES

Benzodiazepines have been around for decades. Temazepam, lormetazepam and loprazolam are the main examples used as hypnotics. They are effective and the dose is short lived, so they have little 'hangover effect'. Nitrazepam, flunitrazepam and flurazepam are all longer lasting, so their effects persist into the next day and tend to build up with repeated doses. They are used less often. Diazepam (Valium) is also long lasting and is not suitable for use as a hypnotic unless there is also a need for relief of daytime anxiety symptoms. Tolerance to all these drugs builds up in two to three weeks, so their effect starts to wane and can lead to the need for a higher dose.

In addition they are addictive and it can be difficult to stop taking them after more than a few weeks because of withdrawal symptoms, which include insomnia. This is said to be more of a problem with the short-acting benzodiazepines but occurs with all of them.

NEWER HYPNOTICS

Zopiclone, zolpidem and zalepon are newer hypnotics, all of them short lasting. The hope that these drugs would be more effective and less prone to causing dependence than the benzodiazepines has not been realised and addiction can still occur.

All of these hypnotic drugs are licensed for 'short-term use only' because of the dependence potential. However, insomnia does not tend to be a short-term problem and the reality is that many people go on to hypnotics and stay on them for months or years. This is a very difficult problem to properly resolve, as one is trying to set off one problem against another. There is no perfect solution, although other types of drug solution do exist and follow shortly. It does not follow that everyone on long-term hypnotics will automatically have problems coming off the drugs, but most do and so it is preferable not to get into this position if possible. This means limiting the use of hypnotics to short spells of two to three weeks maximum and then taking a break for a while. This can maintain the effectiveness of the drug and avoid dependency.

ANTIDEPRESSANTS

The older 'tricyclic' antidepressants like amitriptyline and dothiepin were mentioned in chapter 5 as having sedative properties. As a result they were used a great deal to help depressed patients who had marked sleep problems. However, the sleep they promote is not 'normal' sleep. They do not increase the amount of deep sleep a person has and so while they can help getting off to sleep, they tend not to prevent people still waking in the morning feeling tired.

Most of the newer antidepressants such as the SSRIs are not sedative. They ultimately lead to an improvement in sleep in someone who is depressed by lifting the underlying depression, but this will not necessarily apply in CFS/ME. Mirtazapine and trazodone are relatively new antidepressants which are sedative and they can promote better quality sleep than the tricyclics – trazodone perhaps more so. They also have the advantage of not causing dependency. A low dose of trazodone is therefore an alternative to benzodiazepines.

MELATONIN

Melatonin is a hormone produced by a small part of the brain called the pineal gland and it is thought to be important in regulating sleep behaviour. It is commercially available and is variously classified in different countries as either a food supplement or, as in Europe, as a drug. It is technically possible for a GP to prescribe it in the UK and it is in use as a hypnotic and as a treatment for jet lag. While it may help some people with CFS/ME to sleep it does not have any special effect in the condition. Studies looking at melatonin output in CFS/ME have not shown a deficiency and some actually show an increase, so there is no theoretical basis for using it. It does, however, appear to be safe and to be free of addiction potential.

Chapter 8

Special Groups with CFS/ME

People with severe CFS/ME

The Chief Medical Officer's report makes for disheartening reading on the subject of those people whose condition is severe enough to limit their ability to carry out the ordinary tasks of daily living. As many as 25 per cent of sufferers may be thus affected at some stage in their illness yet these people are quoted as having often felt abandoned by the medical and social services. From the GP's point of view, uncertain perhaps of the validity of the diagnosis, with few tools to hand with which to 'fix' the patient and prevented by time limitations from visiting patients who may be unable to make the journey to the surgery, delivering anything other than a sympathetic ear now and again may be all they feel able to do. The deficiencies in the care of people with severe CFS/ME are clear and acknowledged but the demands on health service resources are many and what is needed is help on the ground.

There is a need for expertise that reinforces and supports the care provided by the primary care team and the social services but which is tuned to the needs of people with CFS/ME. Such services already exist for cancer patients and are very successful. To a much smaller degree they exist for some other equally deserving conditions like diabetes and asthma but for a host of conditions that would benefit from such an arrangement, including CFS/ME, there is no such set-up.

At the moment one can only propose wish lists and hope that they are turned into reality sometime. A geographically wide network of doctors with a special interest in CFS/ME would be very helpful and guidelines for best practice in the care of CFS/ME should be agreed and distributed to Primary Care Organisations, along with the where-withal to make them happen.

CFS/ME in childhood

CFS/ME certainly occurs in children and young people. The younger the person the more alternative possibilities there may be to explain the symptoms but although one does not generally make the diagnosis in children under five years old it could conceivably occur in children younger than that. If CFS/ME in adults has been controversial then in children it has been even more so.

Medical scepticism has been mixed with inappropriate assumptions of children being made ill by over-protective or even deliberately manipulative parents. Lack of understanding in schools can cause major clashes with education authorities and social services can become entangled too when allegations of misguided parental care start flying around.

This perhaps is the worst-case scenario in childhood CFS/ME, and is becoming less common. GPs need good back-up in diagnosing CFS/ME in children, which should always be done in conjunction with a paediatric specialist. Good quality information, understandable to both the child and the family, is essential and needs to feed back also to the school. Flexible learning packages accommodating the child's energy levels reduce the impact of school absence and make it easier to attend, perhaps on a part-time basis. Parents need good advice on financial support, particularly if one has to give up work to become a full-time carer. Families can need support to deal with the altered dynamics that arise when a child has a long-term illness.

Other groups

There is practically no information on the impact of CFS/ME within ethnic groups. The carers of people with CFS/ME are also a neglected group. The CMO's report highlighted the experience of some who have also been subject to poor support from care services. Apart from a need for more research, more practical help in the form of outreach clinics, community-based support nurses and respite care beds are all required to make a significant impact on the consequences of severe CFS/ME.

Moving forward

It would be inappropriate to end this book on a downbeat note, as any discussion on the resource problems of the NHS and social services tends to do. There will probably never be enough money in the pot but at least the fragmentation and under-funding of the care sectors, which characterised the last quarter of the twentieth century, has changed to a more constructive policy in the first few years of the twenty-first. Most important for people with CFS/ME is that the mood has changed and the challenge of this illness is now being taken up in earnest. We can look forward to better days ahead.

Appendix A

References

General

- Shepherd, C.S., and Chaudhuri, A,. 'ME/CFS/PVFS: an exploration of the key clinical issues'; http://www.meassociation.org.uk/meexplo2.pdf
- Murdoch, C., and Denz-Penhey, H., 'Chronic Fatigue Syndrome: a patient-centred approach' (Radcliffe Medical Press, 2002; ISBN 1 85775 9079); http://www.amazon.co.uk/exec/obidos/ASIN/185775 9079
- Fukuda, K., et al., 'The chronic fatigue syndrome: a comprehensive approach to its definition and study' (Annals of Internal Medicine, 1994; 121: 953–9)
- Chaudhuri, A., et al., 'Chronic Fatigue Syndrome (Review)' (Proceedings of the Royal College of Physicians of Edinburgh, 1998; 28: 150–63)

- Marcovitch, H., 'Managing chronic fatigue syndrome in children' (British Medical Journal, 1997; 314: 1635); http://bmj.com/cgi/content/full/314/7095/1635
- Knook, L., 'High nocturnal melatonin in adolescents with chronic fatigue syndrome' (The Journal of Clinical Endocrinology and Metabolism, 2000; 85(10): 3690–2); http://jcem.endojournals.org/cgi/content/full/85/10/3690
- Kavelaars, A., et al., 'Disturbed neuroendocrine-immune reactions in chronic fatigue syndrome' (The Journal of Clinical Endocrinology and Metabolism, 2000; 85(2): 692–6); http://jcem.endojournals.org/cgi/content/full/85/2/692
- Williams, G., et al., 'Therapy of circadian rhythm disorders in chronic fatigue syndrome: no symptomatic improvement with melatonin or phototherapy' (European Journal of Clinical Investigation, 2002; 32(11): 831–7)

Government and other reports

- A report of the CFS/ME Working Group to the Chief Medical Officer, 2002; www.doh.gov.uk/cmo/cfsmereport/index.htm
- Government response to the CFS/ME Independent Working Group's Report, 2002; www.doh.gov.uk/cmo/cfsmereport/response.htm
- 'Chronic Fatigue Syndrome: report of a joint working group of the Royal Colleges of Physicians, Psychiatrists and General Practitioners' (October 1996, revised 1997); http://www.rcplondon.ac.uk/pubs/brochures/pub_print_cfs.htm
- Medical Research Council: CFS/ME Research Advisory Group's draft research strategy for public consultation, December 2002; http://www.mrc.ac.uk/pdf-cfs_consultation_draft_final_version.pdf
- Bagnall, A-M., et al., 'The effectiveness of interventions used in the treatment/management of chronic fatigue syndrome and/or myalgic encephalomyelitis in children and adults' (NHS Centre for Reviews and Dissemination, University of York, 2002); http://www.york.ac.uk/inst/crd/report22.pdf

Exercise

- Fulcher, K.Y., and White, P.D., 'Strength and physiological response to exercise in patients with chronic fatigue syndrome' (Journal of Neurology, Neurosurgery and Psychiatry, 2000; 69: 302–7); http://jnnp.bmjjournals.com/cgi/content/full/69/3/302
- Fulcher, K.Y., and White, P.D., 'Randomised controlled trial of graded exercise inpatients with the chronic fatigue syndrome' (British Medical Journal, 1997; 314: 1647; http://bmj.com/cgi/content/full/314/7095/1647
- Peters, S., et al., 'A randomised controlled trial of groups aerobic exercise in primary care patients with persistent unexplained physical symptoms' (Family Practice, 2002; 19;6: 665–74); http://fampra.oupjournals.org/cgi/content/abstract/19/6/665
- Blackwood, S.K., et al., 'Effects of exercise on cognitive and motor function in chronic fatigue syndrome and depression' (Journal of Neurology, Neurosurgery and Psychiatry, 1998; 65: 541–6); http://jnnp.bmjjournals.com/cgi/content/full/65/4/541

Cognitive behaviour therapy and self-help

- 'Cognitive behaviour therapy for chronic fatigue syndrome' (Bandolier evidence-based medicine archive); http://www.jr2.ox.ac.uk/bandolier/booth/alternat/cbtfatigue.html
- Sharpe, M., et al., 'Cognitive Behaviour Therapy for the chronic fatigue syndrome: a randomised controlled trial' (British Medical Journal, 1996; 312: 22–6); http://bmj.com/cgi/content/full/312/7022/22
- Chalder, T., et al., 'Self-help treatment of chronic fatigue syndrome: a randomised controlled trial' (British Journal of Health Psychology, 1997; 2: 189–97)

Medical opinion

- Stanley, I., et al., 'Doctors and social epidemics: the problem of persistent unexplained physical symptoms, including chronic fatigue' (British Journal of General Practice (editorial), May 2002); www.rcgp.org.uk/rcgp/journal/issues/may02/editor1.asp
- Lloyd, A.R., et al., 'Illness or disease? The case of chronic fatigue syndrome' (Medical Journal of Australia, 2000; 172: 471–2); http://www.mja.com.au/public/issues/172_10_150500/lloyd/lloyd.html

Appendix B

Charities, Support and Professional Organisations

Action for ME

Action for ME
PO Box 1302
Wells
Somerset BA5 1YE

Tel: 01749 670799
Fax: 01749 672561
E-mail: admin@afme.org.uk
Website: http://www.afme.org.uk/index.shtml

ME Association

The ME Association
4 Top Angel
Buckingham Industrial Park
Buckingham
Bucks MK18 1TH

Fax: 01280 821602
Website: http://www.meassociation.org.uk

For the ME Connect and Listening service (available 2–4 and 7–9 p.m. every day of the year, with calls charged at national rate), the appropriate telephone numbers are:

Members only: 08707 442926
Non-members: 0871 7810008

Association of Young People with ME (AYME)

Association of Young People with ME
PO Box 605
Milton Keynes MK2 2XD

Tel: 01908 373300
Fax: 01908 274136
E-mail: info@ayme.org.uk
Website: http://www.ayme.org.uk/index.html

The 25% ME Group

25% ME Group
Douglas Court
Beach Road
Barassie
Troon
Ayrshire KA10 6SQ

E-mail: enquiries@25megroup.org
Website: http://www.btinternet.com/~severeme.group/

Homeopathy

British Homeopathic Association/Faculty of Homeopathy
Tel: 020 7566 7800
Website: http://www.trusthomeopathy.org

Psychology

British Psychological Society
Tel: 0116 2549568
Website: http://www.bps.org.uk

British Association for Behavioural and Cognitive Psychotherapies
Tel: 01254 875277
Website: http://www.babcp.org